Rai

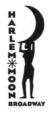

HARLEM MOON

BROADWAY

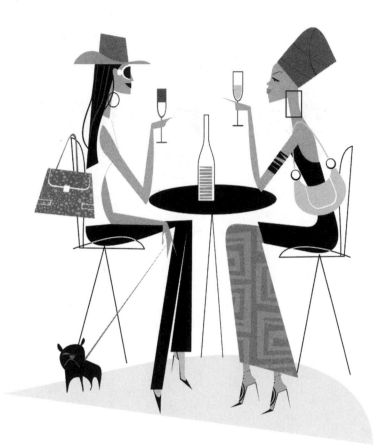

Jenyne M. Raines

Beautylicious!

*The Black Girl's Guide
to the Fabulous Life*

Harlem Moon · Broadway Books
NEW YORK

Published by Harlem Moon, an imprint of
Broadway Books, a division of Random House, Inc.

PRINTED IN THE UNITED STATES OF AMERICA

HARLEM MOON, BROADWAY BOOKS, and the HARLEM
MOON logo, depicting a moon and a woman, are trademarks of
Random House, Inc. The figure in the Harlem Moon logo is
inspired by a graphic design by Aaron Douglas (1899–1979).

Visit our website at www.harlemmoon.com

First edition published 2004.

Book design by Jennifer Ann Daddio
Illustrated by Bee

Library of Congress Cataloging-in-Publication Data
Raines, Jenyne M.
Beautylicious! : the Black girl's guide to the
fabulous life / Jenyne M. Raines.
p. cm.
1. African American women—Health and hygiene.
2. African American teenagers—Health and hygiene.
3. Beauty, Personal.   I. Title.

RA778.4.A36R35 2004
613'.0424'08996073—dc21
2003042339

ISBN 0-7679-1110-5

10 9 8 7 6 5 4 3 2 1

To Jonathan and Carole Raines,
aka Dad and Mom, for being the very best
parents a girl could have and for being supportive
emotionally and financially, especially when
I knew you two were thinking, "The
Board of Ed is hiring . . ."

To my nieces, Kyah Harris and
Shavonne Raines, and my goddaughters,
Shaunna Lewis and Khai Pinkston: The
beautylicious life is yours for the asking!

In memory of my
beautylicious pooch, Kymba

Acknowledgments

y brother and sister, Jason Raines and Stephanie Harris—what a great support system! I love you guys madly. Now a million years later, we see that Dad's strategy of mixing it up at the Apollo, Lincoln Center, and the juke joint down the block made an impression on one of us! Hugs and kisses to Grandma Raines. Smooches to my nephews Steve Jr., Khamaree, and Khenji, bro-in-law Steve, and my relatives!

To the beautylicious babes who put the *b* in buddy and bodaciousness: Kim Singleton, Tina Redwood, Charlotte Hunter, Doris Barry, Ruth Manuel-Logan, Elaine Wallace, Malissa Drayton-Lisbon, Marcita Pinkston, Sheila Parham, Pamela Johnson, Jerilyn Lewis, Robin ("TCB") Whitley, Judy Watson Remy, Danielle Robinson, Erika Kirkland, Frances Bonham, Dawn Baskerville, Jennifer Heslop, Delsi Cunningham, Jackie Reardon, Shawneequa Scott, Karen Halliburton, Linda Johnson, Dina Yassin, Sonya Lockett, Donna Johns, Monique Johnson, Jacklyn Monk, Chrissy Murray, Narine Malcolm, and Karen Jallah.

Muchas gracias to a few guiding lights along the way: Monique Greenwood-Pogue, Susan L. Taylor, Lloyd Boston, Corynne Corbett, Mikki Taylor, Constance White, Patrik Bass, and Patricia M. Hinds.

The Beautylicious Bombshell Squad, aka the experts: Dr. Virgil Hatcher, dermatologist, NYC; makeup pros Roxanna Floyd and Noelle Bonham; Dawn Burrowes, aesthetician, Body

Essential Day Spa, NYC; Barry Fletcher, hairstylist, Avant Garde Hair Gallery, Capital Hills, Maryland; Johnny Gentry, hairstylist, NYC; Derrick Scurry, hairstylist, Brooklyn, NY; Myreah Moore, author and dating guru; Irene Shelley, editor in chief of *Black Beauty and Hair* magazine; Ellen Goldstein, chairperson of the Accessory Design Department at FIT; Tyrone Traylor, hair and makeup; and Dr. Ian Smith. A special thanks to the fabulous females who took the time to share their secrets: Ophelia Devore, Kimora Lee Simmons, Audrey Smaltz, Nicole Narine, Renee Tennison.

Smooches to my editor, Janet Hill, the original beautylicious babe, and her assistant, Tracy Jacobs. J, you were a dream to work with! Smooches also go out to my agent, Charlotte Sheedy, and her assistant, Carolyn Kim, who know what to say to get a girl off the roof, and to Janice K. Bryant for making sure this girl's writing flowed. And of course, a hearty thank you and salute to the patron saints of beautyliciousness: Josephine Baker, A'Lelia Walker, Bricktop, and the Dolls—Lena Horne, Eartha Kitt, Diahann Carroll, Diana Ross, Tina Turner, Grace Jones, and Pam Grier.

Contents

Introduction   *xi*

Chapter One   Queen Me   *3*

Chapter Two   Fit and Fine   *27*

Chapter Three   Soul Power   *49*

Chapter Four   Super Fly   *69*

Chapter Five   Beauty . . . Moi Way   *95*

Chapter Six   Mane Intrigue   *113*

Chapter Seven   Fun and Frolic   *133*

Chapter Eight   Fête Accompli   *153*

Chapter Nine   Date-o-Rama   *167*

Chapter Ten   Luxe Life   *181*

The Fabulous Finale   *203*

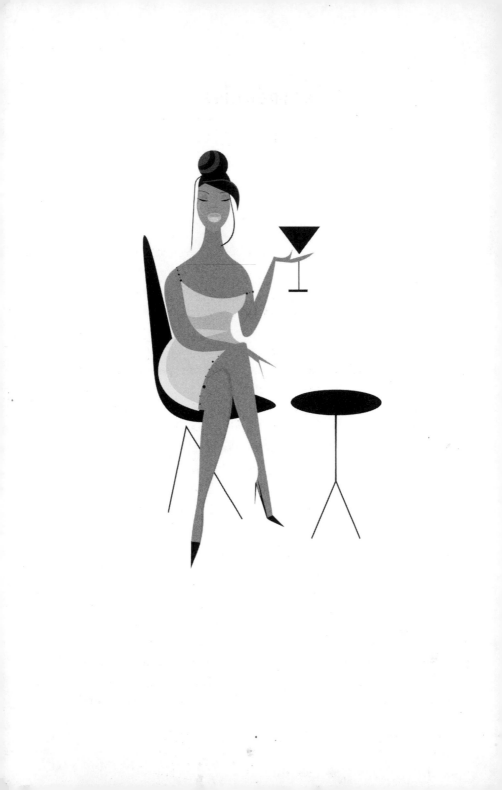

Introduction

HELLO, DOLLFACE!

eautylicious! I know what you're saying: "Damn, give a chick a couple of mojitos, set her in front of a computer, and this is what you get—made-up words and a lot of tomfoolery." Not so, *mon amie.* Beautyliciousness is a way of thinking. It is the place where style, spirit, and funk intersect. It is a celebration of *la vida loca,* joie de vivre, and a whole lotta soul. It's also an instructive mix of contemporary (mis)adventures and (mis)adventurers gleaned from the patron saints of beautyliciousness: Josephine Baker, Bessie Smith, A'Lelia Walker, Madame C. J. Walker, Bricktop, Josephine Premice; and from the luscious living legends affectionately known as the Dolls: Lena Horne! Eartha Kitt! Diahann Carroll! Diana Ross! Tina Turner! Pam Grier! Grace Jones! In other words, anyone with plenty of panache, a dose of derring-do, and who is down for an adventure—street, soigné, or just plain shenanigans.

Before Madonna, who is widely credited with being the queen of style and reinvention, there were the Dolls. Black women with huge dreams and talent. Black women who, with less than two dollars in their chic purse, serve up incredible style and glamour, are world travelers and speak, sing, and cuss in five different languages. The Dolls are the black women who did it their way—by channeling their creativity to get them out of their mundane, often dreary surroundings, educating themselves—through books and exposure—captivating kings and maharajahs and persevering through segregation, racism, and plain ole stupidity. Sisters who were quick with a quip, a bon mot, or a demand, in a time when black women weren't expected to say any more than "Yes ma'am." They are bold, brash, beautiful, and Balenciaga'd down. The new school, which includes Oprah, Mary J. Blige, Halle Berry, Missy Elliott, Macy Gray, Erykah Badu, and others, continues to incite and inspire with their talents, passion, beauty, and indomitable style.

Beautylicious! is a manifesto for going through life with a little swagger, a dash of sauciness, and a lot of grace. Because making things look easy and keeping folks feeling warm and fuzzy is an art, a sister's got to know a trick or five. Tricks like how to keep her hair looking fierce no matter what side of the globe she's on, or how to throw a last-minute shindig on a few pennies and a lot of style, or how to get her mack on in the grocery store. Yep, it's all the stuff your mom didn't teach you because she was more concerned that you become a credit to the race. And beautyliciousness is a reinforcement of Ma's preaching, in such matters as self-esteem, fitness (a must), and your spiritual life, because we all know that without the egg whites the soufflé will fall flat. Think of beautyliciousness as the voice of Aunt Eartha, the ultra-glam aunt who left home to make it in the big city and in the process danced on a few tabletops, sipped champagne with black and white royalty, broke a few hearts, worked the killa dress, and lived life to its grandest—all on her terms!

The beautylicious girl is the bomb, but even a bombshell needs to know how to give Oscar-worthy face, rock a frock, *and* make an entrance that makes the men all pause. The beautylicious gal knows that *extravagant* refers to her spirit *and* her personality, and not necessarily her spending habits. In other words, the beautylicious babe is mad cool. She's down to earth, she's no snob. Simply put, she is witty, smart, and sexy with plenty of nerve and verve to spare. She is diva—hear her laugh!

Beautylicious! The Black Girl's Guide to the Fabulous Life offers shortcuts, tips, and observations on how to live a happy, stylish, authentic life with joy and grace. Now you can get answers to "Don't ask Ma" concerns like how to look sexy the morning after sans the Buckwheat 'do and how to beat a hasty retreat the morning after without offending Brotherman. And because no one, not even the Dolls (well, okay, maybe Diana), is "Showtime at the Apollo" ready 24/7, *Beautylicious!* is also about shoring up your inner beauty so that you can radiate warmth, generosity, and natural elegance even on your worst days! The beautylicious babe celebrates herself but is always kind and loving to others. Healthy self-confidence, supreme self-care, and living the Golden Rule are the true keys to the fabulous life.

But most of all, beautylicious is just a synonym for fun. And that's how you should live your life! So sit back, relax, grab a flute of champagne or sparkling Martinelli's, and enjoy!

Beautylicious!

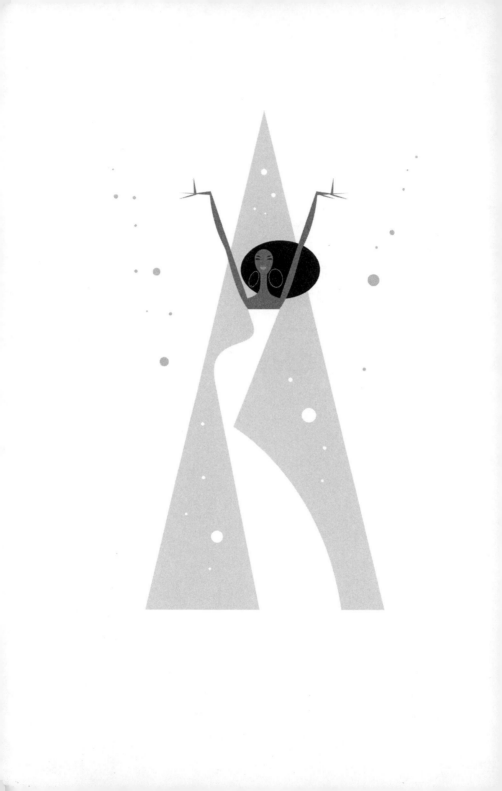

Chapter One

Queen Me

I'm a winner, baby.
—DIANA ROSS, *MAHOGANY*

*L*iterary wit and bon vivant Oscar Wilde said, "To love oneself is the beginning of a lifelong romance." These are the words to live by. This is the bedrock of beauty-liciousness: self-acceptance. Self-acceptance and self-esteem are about being in love with you, about having the ability to truly appreciate your talents, beauty, and uniqueness, and, above all, being comfortable with yourself.

You put the *bomb* in *bombshell.* Your looks are smoldering, your personality is dynamic, and the total you is, well, *kaboom!* Wow! Though you may find yourself asking, "Where is that incendiary minx? Hmm, does she only come out for All Saints Day and the lunar eclipse?" Most of the time you are slinking around like a sweet but meek calico kitty, because you don't quite believe that God's been so good to you. Clearly, you're oblivious to how great you are. You're not alone. The truth is that balancing and maintaining your self-esteem is a lifelong process, one that *no one* is exempt from.

Trust, all of the Dolls, from Josephine Baker to Halle Berry, have had their doubts, doubters, and detractors, but they've also had their hype list, affirmations, goals, and vision. Everyone has had to learn to push past her fears and underlying thoughts of "I'm just an ashy, knock-kneed gal from Harlem" to project "I'm the cat's meow." It may not have been easy; yet they put one Ferragamo-shod foot in front of the other in a soulful strut toward their dream. Sure, you'll fall, but what separates Ms. Beautylicious from the rest of the girls is that she'll get up confident, determined, and laughing. Think of confidence as a verb. It is an action. When you're feeling less than sizzling, do something! It takes an arsenal of mind games, affirmations, and reinforcements to appear confident when you really want to use your head for soccer practice. And, it takes grace, humility, and a bit of humor to recover from life's pratfalls. Don't worry, you'll reclaim the incendiary minx that has always been there. Use the confidence-building tools in your arsenal, but always remember Beautylicious rule number one: *You rule!*

Cast Down Your Buckets

So advised Booker T. Washington in his famous Atlanta conference speech. He was exhorting black folks on how to cope with racism during the turn of the twentieth century. While his advice was, in hindsight, umm, too accommodating of the racial mores of the time, it's right on time for Ms. Beautylicious. Cast down your buckets and pick up your mirror to lovingly assess your unique beauty and to start embracing yourself as you are now. Anyone can think she's ready to take over the world *after* her weave is sewn in or she's dropped twenty pounds, but the base of boomin' beautyliciousness is appreciating what you have now, whether it's your favorite feature or not. When you look in the mirror, know that the person reflected deserves love, fun, loads of fulfilling sex, success, Louis Vuitton bags, and all the best that life has to offer; claim these things and more as your due. And, when a flashback or a bad-hair day has rocked your fab foundation, be sure to reach for your looking glass and *caress* yourself. How? Try this technique, developed by therapist Carolyn

Hillman in her book *Love Your Looks*: Show *Compassion* for whatever you are feeling about yourself, nonjudgmentally. *Accept* yourself and your appearance. *Respect* yourself for who you are. *Encourage* yourself to take the risks and the steps to achieve what you want out of life as you are now. *Support* yourself by believing in yourself and reassuring yourself that how you look is fine. *Stroke* yourself by praising yourself and giving yourself credit for trying. The love fest starts this minute!

Don't Play That Song for Me

What you say to yourself is far more important than what's going on in your life. If the CD *My Greatest Misses and Disses* is on perpetual random play in your head, it limits you—your talents, power, and beauty. How do you stop the litany of negativity? By replacing every negative thought with a positive one. It starts with confronting the negative thought—you know, the "I am fat, I am lazy, I am dumb" conversation that, when you think about it, some small jealous clown from sixth grade bestowed on you and you believed it. Replace that cut in your head with "I am not dumb. I am a smart girl and confident. Hell, I got it going on." The key is you have to say it out loud so that you can get the hang of it and begin to believe it. Repetition is good. Out in public and cut number five, "I am a loser," starts playing? A simple "No," said out loud (but not too loud), believe it or not, helps. It sounds like the last stand against the bogeyman, and in a way it is. *No* makes the offending thoughts dissolve. The real daily deal: Start talking pretty to yourself. Hips are no longer described as humongous. Nope, they're "curvy" and "cushy comfy." Give yourself a shout-out every time you pass the mirror or when a wave of doubt overtakes you. Granted, the first couple of times that you say, "I'd like to say hey to the baddest, smartest babe, I know . . . me!" may crack you up, but it's a great way to quickly shore up your confidence. You can replace the old stale tapes located in the windmills of your mind with a great new one entitled *The Greatest Love of All!*

Fake It Till You Make It

Whether it's interviewing for a new job, giving a speech, or running into your archnemesis while looking less than lovely at the corner bodega, don't let the situation rock your world. Handle it.

Project strength even when you feel shaky. Begin to breathe; take deep breaths, inhaling from the nose, exhaling from the mouth. Shout down that inner voice of self-doubt and visualize yourself as a beautiful woman in control of the situation. There is something to imagining yourself as Condoleeza Rice or any other take-control woman before you give your office presentation. Hell, channel one of your personal best moments: graduation; that particular day that everything was working overtime; or any memory of you feeling great, beautiful, strong, and on top of the world. You'll not only convince others that you are in control but you'll really begin to feel that way. Look at the nervous tics and things you do when your confidence is low. Do you bite your nails, pull on your hair, or talk too fast? Break those habits now. No one will know you're feeling insecure if you don't broadcast it with nervous gestures.

Test Positive

Smell your roses while you're alive. Keep a running tally of your own greatness. Affirm, visualize, and fiercely protect your most exalted self. Here are the tools to help you maintain and bolster your confidence:

THE HYPE REPORT

Picasso dubbed Josephine Baker "the Nefertiti of Now." Orson Welles crowned Eartha Kitt "The Most Exciting Woman in the World." Lofty titles from lofty men, to be sure, but you can bet your Prada that when Jo or Eartha was feeling less than super-starish, those sobriquets cheered them up. Okay, Spike Lee hasn't put your essence into words yet, but I'll wager that your friends, family, and acquaintances have given you accolades. Of course they have, and you should record compliments and stash thank-you notes, letters of achievements, and love letters. Write down what you think is great about you and don't stint on the applause. Have fun with the hype report. List your fabulous traits in a sumptuous silk journal, buy a drawing pad and illus-trate your compliments with cut-up words (from magazines and newspapers) and pictures, or just put together your own press kit, complete with "press clippings," of every glowing mention of you. Write your praises in calligraphy and tape them up to the mirror, where you can see them. Enjoy your external beauty and the manifestations of the internal. Feel free to drag out your list anytime to remind yourself that you are the bomb.

SHINING STAR

> *Baby, you must not be selfish. Let the whole world*
> *benefit from your incredible radiance.*
> —DUKE ELLINGTON

The incomparable Duke said that to Lena Horne. Yes, it's hard to believe that the legendary beauty needed a boost, but it's also another illustration that even the most fabulous of the fabulous don't always think they are the bee's knees. Heed the elegant maestro's statement. You've got something special going on and it's high time the world knew about it! Get out there and share your star power. If you can sing, take it to the stage, to the senior-citizen center, or to your friend's wedding, but don't just save it for the shower. A brilliant mind? Celebrate it, don't dumb down for anyone. Create and teach a course at the local continuing education program. They named you "motor mouth" in seventh grade? Don't hang your head, use your deft verbal skills as an MC. Hey, you can be the next Eve or simply entertain as the mistress of ceremonies for an organization's fashion show. Or volunteer as a publicist for your favorite local haunt. The point is to just celebrate the things that make you you, and do it with your head held high!

THE SUPREME TEAM

Along the road to divadom, all of the Dolls have had to pack the proverbial security blanket along with the sequined gowns in order to quell potentially crippling fears and build sagging confidence. Some blues tools that you can use:

Diana Ross believes in positive thinking tapes. "One of my greatest tools has been my positive thinking tapes. I use them constantly; they are a great source of inspiration, and I'm not embarrassed to let people know how much they inspire and assist me in maintaining my self-esteem."

Kimora Lee Simmons looks inward. "When my confidence is kind of low, I do whatever I have to do to make myself feel better. It may be a yoga class, a warm bath, or writing in my journal—anything that makes me peaceful, because I can do great work when I am peaceful."

Josephine Premice gazes into the looking glass. "I got over thinking I was ugly. A friend told me to stand in front of the bathroom mirror and repeat over and over, 'I am beautiful.' It worked. I began to feel beautiful, which is very important."

Mary J. Blige finds solace in the Bible. "I realized that my life was a gift from God and if I did not take responsibility for saving myself nobody else would."

My Life: The Remix

I don't lie. I improve on life.
—JOSEPHINE BAKER

Our girl Jo may have been the original mix master, for she gleefully rewrote and reinvented her life at will. One guess is it was

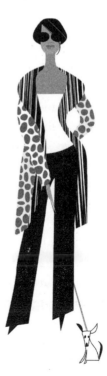

partially to keep a sad and painful background hidden, and then after a while she did it simply because she could! The fab girl goes with a more modern, shall we say P. Diddyish, way of looking at her life. There is your life story, the pain, the glory, and the yawn of it. And there's the remix, which is used for the rest of the world. Now when I say remix, I don't mean outrageous lies. If you come from Baldwin Hills with two perfectly respectable accountants for parents, you don't tell people you're an orphaned princess from Tanzania who joined the circus. Save that for your creative writing course. I mean you are free to spin events that are not comfortable for you or no one's business in a manner that makes you feel empowered. You don't owe anyone and everyone full disclosure that you've taken the bar exam fifteen times or that you've revisited Bob, a poor choice for a boyfriend, fifteen times. The only exception to this rule is your physician. Ten to one, your parents don't need to know that you, ahem, were a party girl at college. Your doctor, however, does. Leave whatever you feel doesn't empower you at home. Psychologically this helps you, as you are not forced to relive a painful event, or dwell on what you perceive as a failure. For instance, while there is no shame in being fired—it happens to most people at one time or another—you don't need to give a potential employer or your ex–office mate the low-down dirty version. If your response is: "Mr. Jones/Girlfriend, I had to go 'cause my boss was a jealous, hateful shrew who always picked on me. I mean, gosh, so I came in late a couple of times and didn't do the proposal she was supposed to write, that heifer didn't have to do what she did . . ." Check the remix: "No, I am no longer at Acme, it really wasn't a fit." Notice how the remix kills all of the negatives; you're not going back down memory lane about your boss nor are you planting any negative impressions about yourself or your work habits in someone else's mind. And you told the truth; you're not working at Acme anymore. There is no rule saying that the assorted and sundry people you meet in life have to know everything. You choose who gets the privilege of knowing you inside and out.

Personal Courage

To most of us, one of the highest compliments, yet a faintly damning insult, is "You're such a nice girl." Yes, we all want to be seen as that wonderful gal who bakes cookies, supplies friends with both shoulders and Kleenex to cry on, forgives the love man's major transgressions, gives her last dollar to the homeless, and leaps from tall buildings in a single bound. Er, sure, most days you're like that, but every now and again you just want to be left alone to do your own thing, give Brotherman and the selfish friend the tongue-lashing they deserve, and, well, spend a little time with your less-than-saintly side. How do you tell people where to go and how to get there, or just tell them, "No, I prefer to clean out the fuzz in my belly button"? Lightbulb moment: Just say *"No!"* The word *no* should be used freely, especially if it is going to protect your feelings, safety, and sanity.

Manners Make the Babe

We're training them for Buckingham Palace and the White House.
—MAXINE POWELL

So decreed the Supremes' etiquette coach, referring to the endless poise, diction, and etiquette classes the singular girl group had to take. Hmm, now there's a quaint notion. Why would anyone need training in the new millennium? Baby, it's a Barnum and Bailey world. Jerry Springer antics, shot caller/baller/brawler mentality, and general ignorance seem to be the norm in all levels of society, while it appears that such qualities as poise, civility, and respect for oneself and others have gone the way of the Afro Sheen Blowout Kit. The beautylicious babe keeps it real by upholding the social graces, because she knows that good manners are the universal language. We all could brush up on matters of deportment, so I went old school for pointers from the mighty trinity of black finishing-school divas: Ophelia DeVore of Ophelia DeVore's School of Charm, New York City; Maxine Powell of Maxine Powell's Model, Host and Hostess Agency and Motown Records in Detroit; and Charlotte Hawkins Brown, educator and founder of Palmer Memorial Institute in Sedalia, North Carolina.

Now sit up straight and absorb what they have to say.

CHARMED

The Doyenne of Charm, Ophelia DeVore, worked with the Dolls Diahann Carroll, Attalah Shabazz, Cicely Tyson, style diva Audrey Smaltz, and *Essence* editorial director Susan Taylor. Here she lays down the law on how to be more captivating and defines that elusive quality called charm.

J.R. : What is charm?

Ms. DeVore: Charm is a magical force of unlimited, positive energy, originating deep within, reflecting our purest characteristics, which can attract and endear others to us. Charm includes our finest qualities—physical, mental, and spiritual, and when applied unselfishly can fuel positive growth. Essentially, charm is the magnet of persuasion. It compels maximum interest, attention, admiration; it's the ability to bring the best of us to the surface.

J.R. : How does one go about cultivating charm?

Ms. DeVore: Everyone is born with charm! However, if you don't use it, you lose it. Constantly develop the best in yourself and extend that same type of effort to help others to reach their maximum enlightened self-interest. Communications skills are essential, for they allow one's most effective presentation to take the spotlight at all times.

J.R. : What would you like to impart to the Sisters about poise and charm?

Ms. DeVore: As best you can, remove all negative

thoughts and influences from you and your environment. Get rid of the chips on your shoulder by not blaming or resenting others for failure, put your best foot forward, and think only about what you can and will do. *You* control your destiny. Have confidence in yourself and go for the things that you feel passionate about. Continue your education, for you can enhance your confidence by learning many diverse skills. Maintain a network of supportive, quality relationships, which foster high ideals and profound growth.

J.R. : How do I shore up my confidence?
Ms. DeVore: Take responsibility and be accountable. Continue to learn and achieve more effectively. Discover new experiences. Shed old negative baggage that will hold you back. Do what you know to be the right thing.

J.R. : How important is posture?
Ms. DeVore: Good posture is vital; it immediately defines who you are and establishes your visual image. Remember, hold your head high and look everybody in the eye. Practice better posture with the book-on-the-head exercise. Walk and sit with a straight back, walk tall with your head high in a level position as if the top of your head were touching the ceiling and your chin parallel to the floor. Feet should be pointed straight forward with arms rounded to the side. Add a positive attitude and happy thoughts and a smile on your face and in your eyes.

J.R. : Thank you, Ms. DeVore.
Ms. DeVore: I just want the girls to remember this one thing: You came into this world almost perfect and free as the breeze. Don't stray too far away from your birthright.

> *Q:* What phrase is timeless and chic yet very underutilized?
>
> *A:* Thank you
>
> *Q:* What gesture coupled with *thank you* serves as a magic carpet to bigger and better things?
>
> *A:* A smile

CLASS IS IN SESSION

Today the idea of class is treated like an archaic notion relegated to the far reaches of Grandma's attic along with her velvet portrait of Abraham, Martin, and John. Ms. Beautylicious knows that class—which simply is relating to, and interacting with, people in a thoughtful manner—is a learned response and not an inherited trait. Or one predicated on social status. As one can see by the newspapers, any televised award show, and *E! The True Hollywood Story*, money, fame, beauty, and birthright are no indicators of class. Afraid that your manners are on a par with those of Anna Nicole Smith? Not to worry, the beautylicious babe need only employ the tenets of ladyhood, as outlined by educator and founder of the prestigious Palmer Memorial Institute in North Carolina, Charlotte Hawkins Brown. Brown, the grandaunt of Natalie Cole, was well known for turning out polished, poised, and well-versed ladies back in the day.

Twelve Earmarks of a Lady

A LADY

1. Is polite when entering or leaving a room. *Twenty-first-Century Breakdown:* Acknowledge your fellow man's

presence on the planet with a smile and a hello, in
general, but especially in close quarters.

2. Graciously answers, "Yes, Miss A," when called or "No,
   Mrs. B" should the reply require such. *Twenty-first-
   Century Breakdown:* Neither your mother nor your friends
   nor your boss is interested in being addressed with "Yo,"
   "What," or "Huh."

3. Uses "Please," "Thank you," "Excuse me," "Good
   morning," and "Good-bye" as part of her daily speech.

4. Does not chew gum in public. *Twenty-first-Century
   Breakdown:* Chews gum with mouth closed. Knows to
   ditch gum when involved in a conversation, interview, or
   when accepting an award.

5. Awaits her turn; never brusquely pushes ahead. Er, today
   this one is a matter of survival, to avoid a beatdown.

6. Plays fair and works fair.

7. Does not take things that belong to another. *Twenty-first-
   Century Breakdown:* You'd be surprised at the lack of
   comprehension of this concept.

8. Avoids loud and boisterous laughter and conversation.
   Twenty-first-Century Breakdown: The folks on the bus or
   in the supermarket line are not interested in a recap of
   your madcap antics with Latrell or your drunken take on
   world events. Keep it down, Toots.

9. Does not laugh at the mistakes or misfortunes of others.
   Twenty-first-Century Breakdown: Try! Try! Try!

10. Develops a clear, resonant voice and is able to speak well,
    enunciate clearly, pronounce words correctly, and talk
    interestingly of the subjects of the day. *Twenty-first-
    Century Breakdown:* Let's cut the politically correct
    nonsense. With the sorry exception of rappers
    and ballplayers, you will never go far on Ebonics,
    for shizzell!

11. Does not talk constantly about herself. *Twenty-first-Century Breakdown:* Self-explanatory. A boor is a bore.

12. Isn't a killjoy. Uses tact. *Twenty-first-Century Breakdown:* Refrain from making mean-spirited or hurtful comments under the guise of telling the truth. Understand that nine out of ten times it is *your* truth, based on your experiences, perspective, and reality, and it probably won't serve the person it was meant to "help." Think before you speak.

SIT TIGHT, SIT RIGHT

Glide like a swan into your seat. Maxine Powell, the legendary grooming guru at Motown (when it was Hitsville USA), tells you how:

+ Approach the chair at an angle.
+ Touch the seat with the inside leg and put one foot forward.
+ Slide in gracefully and then cross your ankles.
+ Put your feet flat on the floor and make sure your rear is three inches from the back of the chair.

Sure, there'll be a few jeers from the less enlightened. And you'll hear a few seventh-grade refrains like "She thinks she's cute" or "She's stuck-up." But remember this from the annals of junior high: The "snooty" girl always had everyone's respect and the boys always treated her a bit differently. Give it a try.

The Queen of Soul says it best: *R-E-S-P-E-C-T.* Respect is the linchpin of the power of C: Confidence, Charm, and Class. Respect yourself, your elders, those around you, the life of all creatures big and small, the lesson in any situation, and you will be the ultimate class act.

Team Me

Psst ... I'll let you in on a little secret that is sure to free your mind. Jada Pinkett Smith, Halle Berry, and all the other high-wattage vixens didn't just emerge from the Planet Fine looking beautiful with signature hairdo and Versace wardrobe in place. The Girls have an army of people—stylists, makeup artists, hairdressers, manicurists ... I could go on, but you get it—to help create their looks. Now of course, their personal battalion of pros are working with lovely raw material, but work still has to be done! The beautylicious babe's rockin' move? Get your own beauty team going. Just knowing that you have professionals dedicated to keeping you at your finest is a real confidence booster. First you need to determine what the best you should look like. To get the team started, begin with these few simple exercises.

- ✦ Clip mags for your favorite hairdo, clothing, jewelry, and accessories.
- ✦ Make a list of your personal health and beauty goals, i.e., "I want to lose five pounds" or "I want to clear up my skin."
- ✦ Create a personal beauty journal and file the information, as well as the steps you need to take and have taken to meet your goal.

Great. You have a clear idea where you want to go with your looks. Next you want to put your all-star lineup of experts together. Here's the list of those you must have to fire up your beautyliciousness:

1. Hairstylist
2. Nail technician
3. Stylist, either a fashion-savvy friend whose taste and opinion you trust or a favorite saleswoman at your favorite department store
4. Aesthetician
5. Dermatologist. Persistent acne, uneven skin tone, and hair loss are all the provinces of the skin doctor.
6. Gynecologist. Duh! If the plumbing's foul, who cares about the rest of the package?
7. Makeup artist. Of course you sit at the mirror and play around with your own look, but you can find a great makeup artist at the department store. Check out the work at a couple of counters and get your face beat. Like what you see? Make friends, get a card, and find out if she does makeup in her free time and what it costs. Smart money says cough up the dough to get a lesson on a basic look and then keep her on hand for special events.
8. Tailor. The key to making your clothes look like they've been created just for you is through alteration. And a really good tailor can create some basic garments for you.
9. Dentist. Someone's got to keep those pearly whites white, straight, and healthy.
10. Internist. None of this "I am scared of the doctor" nonsense. You should have a physical examination every year. And you should feel comfortable with your doctor, so that you can point out every little twinge and ache that you have, as well as ask questions when you don't understand something. When I don't understand the

medical lingo, I like to say,
"Excuse me, Dr. Jones, I wasn't
sitting behind you in class at
med school, so I am afraid
you'll have to break that down
into layman's terms for me." If
he or she doesn't laugh, or
more important, doesn't
explain it until you get it, find
another doctor.

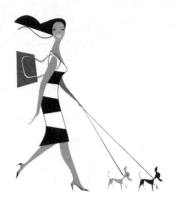

11. Personal trainer. He doesn't necessarily have to come from
the chichi health club. Again, this can be a friend who's a
physical fitness buff.

Team Me, ideally, is a cohesive unit. For example, your hairstylist and dermatologist should be of one accord about the health
of your hair. Any breakage or the use of any medicine should be
common knowledge to both professionals. As the client you also
want to make sure everyone is clear about your goal, which is
the Three Fs—Fit, Fine, and Fabulous!

Shrink Rap

> *I became convinced that my mother's original*
> *advice—to seek professional help when I'm hurting—*
> *was something I should never doubt and to*
> *hell with anyone's objection.*
> —HALLE BERRY

There are times in every beautylicious babe's life when she
realizes that sympathetic friends and a tub of Ben & Jerry's
Chunky Monkey ice cream aren't enough to get her through a

particularly rough spot. The roughest spots, believe it or not, are not when the boyfriend dumps you or you hear the devastating news that that cute Dior T-shirt was a limited edition and is no

The Twinkie Theorem

BEAUTYLICIOUS BELIEF: You can always find money or at least a way to get what you truly need. I came to that conclusion one day when I was dead broke (probably yesterday) and I had a real yen for a Twinkie (aka nonessential "food" item). I started with my wallet, which had lint in it, and then proceeded to tear the apartment up until I found a dollar for this ohh-so-necessary snack. Needless to say, after rolling on the floor looking under the bed and the rugs and in the corners of the cabinet, I discovered some change. Mission accomplished. The next time the goal was a big-ticket item. I couldn't live without a Louis Vuitton bucket bag (yes, technically it's considered nonessential). Again, lint in the wallet, cobwebs in the bank account. Hold on! A bit of credit left on the charge card and a couple of dollars (all right, hundreds) from the rent money and voilà, Louis and I are back together again. And yes, by some stroke of fate, I was able to pay the rent. The Twinkie Theorem is simply an illustration of what happens when you decide that you have to have something and you're willing to step out on faith. Or as the Scripture says, "Now faith is the substance of things hoped for, the evidence of things not seen," Hebrews 11:1.

> The moral of my story is that if you can find money for Twinkies, or the latest designer bag, you must use your powers for good health.

longer in stock, but when you keep going down the same dead-end alley looking for a different result. Replaying negative past experiences prevent you from fully enjoying your life. What exactly does that look like?

The best example is when the need to have a boyfriend becomes so overwhelming that you're throwing yourself on the most inappropriate guys (read druggies, deadbeats, and otherwise attached bros), and they have the nerve to be choosy about you. You're crazed, you're twisting yourself into a pretzel to get loser boy to lavish a bit of attention on you, and you're making yourself and everyone around you a little frightened about your mental health.

Those are the warning signs that it's time to sit down. (For a full list of warning signs, see Couch Bound, page 24.) I mean it. Retreat to your bedroom and really feel your emotions. Write them down. Get quiet. Chances are you'll find that your actions aren't about the lack of a boyfriend but that you're running from something else. Didn't get that far in your self-discovery or don't know what to do now that you have looked within? Enlist the help of a mental health practitioner. Yep, look into therapy.

Black people traditionally have scoffed at counseling. Our motto: No emotional problem is so big that alcohol, drugs, Oprah, or the church can't solve it. Therapy is for the crazy and the rich white folks. No, dear. Therapy is for those who have an issue that they cannot cope with or those who would like to know why and what in their thought process is holding them back from living their most fabulous, purposeful life. Therapy is about excavating to discover the cause and/or root of a habit or a problem with the help of a compassionate, nonjudgmental ear. If you need a professional to listen to you and help you sort things out, by all means get one. Need a nudge? Read *Broken Silence: Black Women in Therapy* by Dr. D. Kim Singleton. And don't worry about cost. (See The Twinkie Theorem, page 22). And you can always ask about sliding-scale payment.

Ask friends and your doctor for referrals or contact the American Psychological Association, www.apa.org, (800) 964–2000, or the Association of Black Psychologists, www.abpsi.org, and ask them to recommend a mental health expert in your area.

COUCH BOUND

Ten signs you may need to lie down: If you can't seem to boost your level of self-esteem or if your actions are self-destructive, you should consider seeking professional treatment. A therapist is a neutral person, an objective ear, unlike a friend or family member who is restraining him- or herself (sometimes) from giving an opinion. Balancing and maintaining your self-esteem, and quite honestly, your sanity, is a lifelong process, one that sometimes requires help. Again, don't be ashamed; most of the Dolls have sought out the help of a therapist. If you exhibit any of the following symptoms, pick up the phone and book an hour with a professional.

1. Inability to cope with problems and daily activities
2. Constant seeking of approval from family, friends, and coworkers
3. Excessive anxieties
4. Prolonged depression and apathy

5. Inability to sleep at least seven and a half hours at night without a sleep aid
6. Extreme mood swings, high or low
7. Abusing alcohol, drugs, sex, or even food
8. Focusing on your faults, whether real or imagined
9. Experiencing a paralyzing sense of dread in social situations
10. Loss of interest in activities that previously provided pleasure

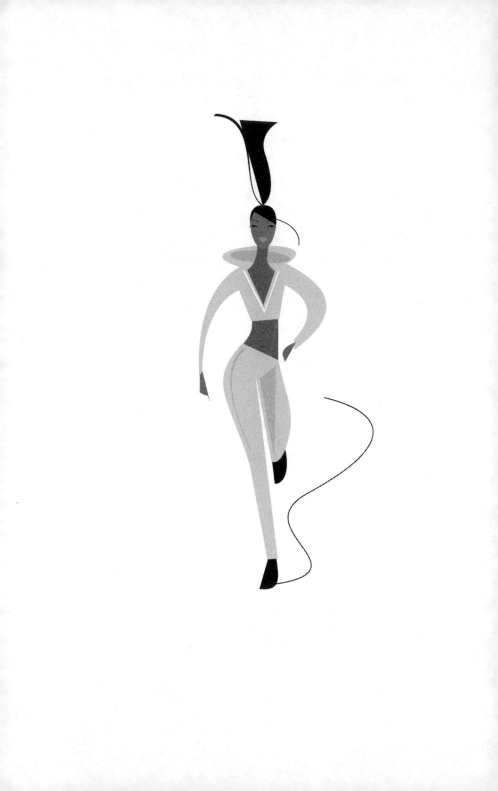

Chapter Two

Fit and Fine

*I am about being healthy. And according
to my doctor I can be healthy at two
hundred pounds. I'm also about feeling
good at whatever size I am.*
—QUEEN LATIFAH

"You've got to love yourself and do the work to sustain your most powerful engine: good health. Without it nothing else matters," opines beautylicious icon Oprah Winfrey. The most valuable instrument you can ever own is a healthy and fit body. Yet we treat this precious vessel so cavalierly, with indiscriminate eating, little or no movement, and a "no-time" approach to our health. Is it any wonder that we black women are more at risk of developing diabetes, cardiovascular disease, and hypertension? We all know what we have to do to keep looking and feeling our best, but honestly, who wants to put in the time or sweat equity of exercise, or give money to the doctor when you know you feel fine? Reflect on what The O said. It's time to love yourself up, not in the form of a new Gucci top, but by cutting back on your Krispy Kreme jones and adding twenty minutes of walking to your day. I won't bore you with a litany of diets or exercises. Naw, that's not the beautylicious way; instead we're going to uncover playful ways to jumpstart your attitude toward exercise, doctors, and diets, and get you jazzed enough to create your own blueprint for good health. You can start by tossing your beliefs and fears. Examine your motivation. As the supa dupa fly Missy Elliott warns, "If you're struggling to lose weight, just make sure it's not because the world wants you to. If it's for health reasons, great." Trust, trying to please everyone but yourself gets old quickly. Also, don't hesitate to use the Dolls as your inspiration. They're still fierce, with bodies that don't look a day over thirty. They're also vital and active. No, it's not the genes or plastic surgery as much as an ongoing commitment to themselves, which includes diet and exercise. Check it out: Pam's curves are still dangerous at fifty, Tina's still hot legs at sixtyish, and Eartha . . . well, that one is in fine feline form, doing handstands at seventyish. And in Pam's case, exercise and healthy eating helped her beat cancer. Take your cue from the Godfather of Soul: Get up! Get into it, and get involved! Let that be your mantra. Okay, now that you're stoked to get the heart pumpin' and the body bumpin', it's time to (if you haven't already) establish a relationship with a cadre of medical professionals. As Ma always said, you can't take good health for granted. Partner with your physician so that you can keep close tabs on your body's functions. Ms. Beautylicious has a clear mandate to take care of herself, for the world needs her laughter and her smile!

The Doctor Is In

Black folks have a tendency to shy away from going to the doctor. Yes, we all have friends who treat themselves like a stray dog. Instead of eating grass and baying piteously when they're not feeling well, they reach for that wonder drug, a can of ginger ale. After downing the Schweppes they continue to carry on about how some body part hurts, but with the love of the Lord and ginger ale, by golly, they'll get through it. What a drag! Oops! Perhaps that's you.

Well, let's call it what it is. If you're scared, ask your friends and family if they can recommend a doctor. Or ask your friend to take you to her doctor. In other words, don't be a scaredy cat. The beautylicious babe makes her visits to the doctor a positive experience. She acts just as she would if she were going to a spa. It's time for your annual checkup? Take a day off and declare it My Health Day. Schedule the internist, gynecologist, and maybe a third doctor (depending on locations and traveling time) about two hours apart. At the end of your visits treat yourself to a great lunch or dinner, as well as some pampering, like a manicure, massage, or lacy bra-and-panty set. Assuming the position in the gyn's office doesn't seem so daunting, does it?

MA! I'VE GOT A DATE WITH A DOCTOR!

Get out that Palm Pilot or Kate Spade date book and make some health dates for yourself. Medical experts recommend scheduling the following appointments for preventive care. Of course, if you have a medical condition or a family history of certain diseases, talk to your doctor about the appointment plan that's right for you. Think of this as your RSVP to good health. Below are your invites to a healthier, more empowered you!

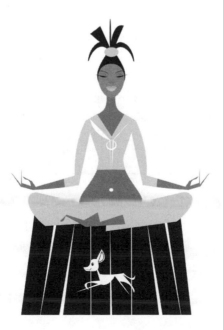

Who:
Primary care physician, aka the internist

What:
Monitors your general health. Checkups should include blood pressure readings and a fecal occult blood test to screen for problems such as inflammatory bowel disease and colon cancer.

When:
Once a year

Special notes:
Get a fasting blood sugar test every two years to screen for diabetes. And if you're in your thirties or over, get a cholesterol screening (every five years, if things are cool). This is a must, especially if you're at increased risk for heart disease because of smoking, family history, obesity, high blood pressure, or diabetes.

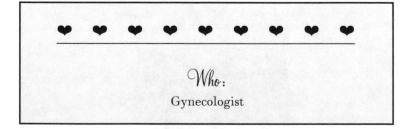

Who:
Gynecologist

What:

Monitors your reproductive health. Checkup should include a Pap smear, pelvic exam, clinical breast exam, and if you're sexually active, screening for sexually transmitted diseases and HIV/AIDS.

When:

Once a year

Special notes:

If you get around (in the Biblical sense), get a Pap smear and STD test every six months.

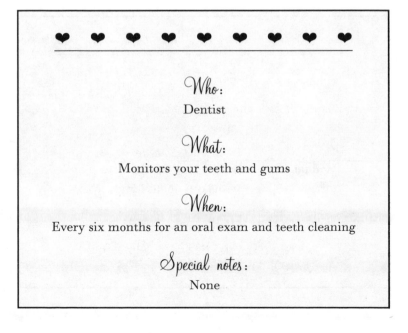

Who:

Dentist

What:

Monitors your teeth and gums

When:

Every six months for an oral exam and teeth cleaning

Special notes:

None

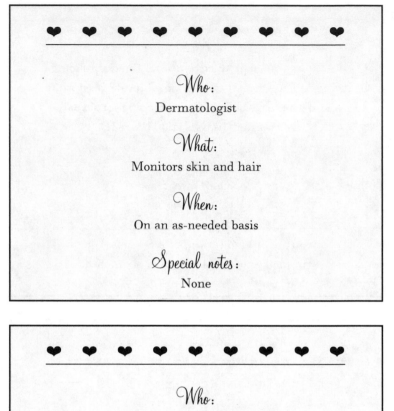

Who:
Dermatologist

What:
Monitors skin and hair

When:
On an as-needed basis

Special notes:
None

Who:
Ophthalmologist

What:
Monitors your eyes. The visit should include an
intraocular pressure measurement for glaucoma.

When:
At least every two years (especially if you
wear glasses). When you hit sixty-five go annually.

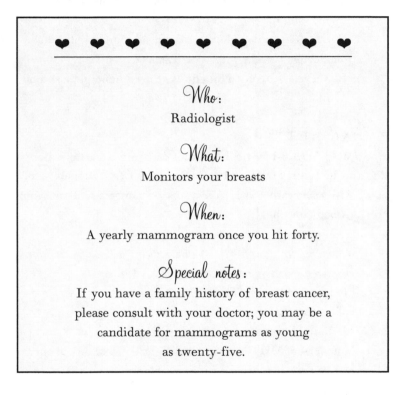

Special notes:
None

Who:
Radiologist

What:
Monitors your breasts

When:
A yearly mammogram once you hit forty.

Special notes:
If you have a family history of breast cancer,
please consult with your doctor; you may be a
candidate for mammograms as young
as twenty-five.

WHAT'S UP, DOC?

Five tactics to help you get the best medical attention. Remember,
it's your health, so be vigilant. Be vocal.

1. Before you visit the doctor, prepare a list of questions in writing.
2. Don't leave the medical appointment until all of your questions have been answered.
3. Bring a list of all the medications you're taking and the dosages, including herbal remedies, vitamins, and over-the-counter drugs.
4. When seeing a new doctor, call ahead to make sure the old doctor has sent your records ahead.
5. If you're discussing a diagnosis or treatment, get a second opinion.

PAGING MD INFO

You should have a few health tomes on your bookshelf alongside the E. Lynn Harris collection. These Beautylicious selections will cover any basic questions or concerns about your precious body and health:

Our Bodies Ourselves for the New Century. A Book by and for Women, Boston Women's Health Book Collective (Touchstone Books). The definitive guide on women's bodies and their reproductive health.

What Your Mother Never Told You About Sex, Hilda Hutcherson, MD (Putnam Publishing). Frank talk about how to make sex safe and pleasurable from one of the nation's top ob-gyns, because you shouldn't be getting the bulk of your sex ed from your friend Fast-Tail Annie or Bishop Don Magic Juan.

Women's Bodies, Women's Wisdom, Christiane Northrup (Bantam Books). A brilliant book that looks at how your emotional well-being, and lack thereof, can be reflected on your gynecological health. Bet you never thought that the recurring yeast infection was your body's way of telling you to show Omar the door.

The Merck Manual of Medical Information: Home Edition, Robert Berkow (Pocket Books); or *Harvard Medical School Family Health Guide,* Anthony L. Komaroff (Simon & Schuster). Each is a compendium of symptoms and diseases. Great for determining possible illnesses and at-home treatments as well as first-aid info. They also help you better communicate with your doctor.

Heal Thyself (A&B Book Publishing); and *Sacred Woman: A Guide to Healing the Feminine Body, Mind and Spirit* (One World Publishing), both by Queen Afua. Guide to relating to your body, health, and emotions from a holistic Afrocentric standpoint.

Brown Skin: Dr. Susan Taylor's Prescription for Flawless Skin, Hair and Nails, Susan C. Taylor, MD (Amistad). An immensely readable manual that offers women of color valuable information and prevention and treatment strategies on caring for our skin, hair, and nails.

Also bookmark these websites: Great for explanations of various illnesses, webmd.com also gives the lowdown on over-the-counter drugs, as in what they are, what they do, and (probably most important) their compatibility with food, drink, and other drugs. The site goaskalice.com offers solid medical advice and thoughtful answers on questions pertaining to your sexual health.

Roots: A Medical Story

Another way to be proactive about your health is to arm yourself and your doctor with information about your family. Grab a notepad and start grilling everyone who will talk. You need to know who has suffered serious diseases—from high blood pressure, diabetes, and cancer to mental illness—so that your physician can best determine which diseases you are predisposed to because of genetics or environment.

TIME TO DRAW UP A NEW FAMILY HEALTH TREE?

+ Collect information on three generations: grandparents, parents, and your own generation, including all brothers and sisters.
+ Write down any major illness of each of your kin.
+ Take note of the age the disease struck, if the relatives are deceased, jot down their ages when they died. Include info on their lifestyles and occupations. This is no time to be coy or judgmental: If Grandpa was a hard drinker who worked off and on at the steel mill, call it. Did your people smoke or work around toxic chemicals?
+ Ask Mom: (A) At what age did she get her period? (B) At what age did she first get pregnant, and was the pregnancy difficult? (C) Does she have fibroid tumors? (D) Did she have them treated? If so how? (E) At what age did she go through menopause?

Let's Take the Die Out of Diet

Listen, I know that a life without Krispy Kreme doughnuts and fried chicken is a life not worth living. I am in total agreement. However, a life with less refined sugar, fats, and fried food will be healthier and longer. The goal is to eat healthy at least 80 percent of the time. Limit your favorite pig-outs (barring a health problem) to 20 percent of the time or schedule one once a week.

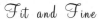

THE DOCTOR WEIGHS IN

Nothing adds gravity and an air of seriousness to a discussion like the input of (drumroll please) a physician. And guess what? If you won't go to him, I will bring him to you. A word from our beautylicious pal, network television news medical expert, author, and devastatingly charming Dr. Ian Smith:

+ Exercise four to five days a week for forty-five minutes with at least one day focusing on weight training.
+ Increase fruits and vegetables in your diet and lower (but don't eliminate) fat intake.
+ Spend at least thirty minutes every day participating in a relaxing activity of leisure—whether reading a book, meditating, or listening to music you enjoy.
+ Clean out your medicine cabinet yearly and review all of your prescriptions with your physician to make sure you still need to be on certain medications and that the dosages and frequency are still valid.
+ Avoid long periods of inactivity, whether at home or at work. The body is best maintained by movement, not sitting still.
+ Don't consume or use herbal supplements before checking with your physician to find out the potential effects and side effects. Cross-reactions can occur between prescribed medications and herbal supplements, so getting the okay before using them can be critical to your health.

WHAT YOU CAN DO RIGHT THIS MINUTE

Oh, a diet can be so daunting. But you can take a few baby steps that add up to big calorie losses!

Say no to soda. A twelve-ounce can of soda can pack 120

calories. Go with my motto of "I'd rather eat my calories" and you'll find yourself sipping on water and diet sodas, both of which have no calories.

Skip the chips. Having an attack of the crunchies? Instead of reaching for the potato chips, especially from the ninety-nine-cent bag, which adds at least five hundred calories and seventeen grams of fat mostly to your thighs, reach for pretzels, which have little to no fat.

Eat your citrus, don't slurp it. Downing a glass of orange juice is a quick way to load up on calories. Instead, eat an orange and save sixty calories per day, and it will keep you feeling fuller longer.

Substitute condiments. Substitutions that won't assault your taste buds and have few to no calories: *mustard* instead of mayo on turkey sandwiches; *salsa* or *hot sauce* on the baked potato instead of butter. If you must dip into the bread basket, go Italian and ask for *olive oil* instead of butter.

BEAUTYLICIOUS BELIEF: Not that I am on his payroll (although I'd like to be!), I must say that George Foreman's Grill is the handy-dandiest product going. It has made eating and cooking healthier a delicious experience. Marinate your skinned chicken, salmon, or tuna steaks for at least thirty minutes in a mixture of low sodium soy sauce, olive oil, and assorted seasonings; throw the food on the grill; and voilà, seven (fish) to twenty (chicken, depending on piece) minutes later you're chowing down on a tasty piece of protein. You don't even miss the fact that it's not fried or strangled by sauce. The bonus? The grill is a cinch to clean!

The healthiest fast-food choices, according to the Center for Science in the Public Interest:

Wendy's Mandarin Chicken Salad

Burger King Chicken Whopper Jr. (or any grilled chicken sandwich—tell them to hold the mayo)

Subway's Select Subs—The idea is to load up on the veggie fixin's and to bypass the mayo and cheese.

Pizza—Make sure it's a thin crust and loaded with veggies for added benefits. Also get in the habit of blotting the oil on the pizza with a napkin and you'll slash about forty-five extra calories.

Diet, shmiet. I'm not going into the pros and cons of the Atkins diet or Sugar Busters; that's what the media's for. Why don't you create an eating plan that you can stick to for the next sixty years? We all know the basics for a healthy body. Make veggies, fruits, and unsaturated oils the basis of your meals, with protein, preferably fish or fowl, as an accompaniment. Eat in moderation; that means no more sides of beef masquerading as steak—a serving of meat should be the size of the palm of your hand. A good habit to get into when dining out? Halve your entrée and put the rest in a doggie bag before you start eating. Once the food is packed up, no matter how ravenous you are, your good upbringing will keep you from going into the bag for more.

Need help with designing an eating and fitness plan? Well, there is no shortage of books on the market, but two that do a really nice job of helping you look at the emotional component of getting fit are *8 Minutes in the Morning: A Simple Way to Burn Fat in 4 Weeks* by Jorge Cruise (HarperResource), and *Get With the Program* by Bob Greene (Simon & Schuster).

AGUA, POR FAVOR

Simple H_2O is the nectar from the gods, but it never seems to have a chance next to a Big Gulp full of cola. Too bad, because water is essential to our health. We cannot exist without it. It is the most important thing we put in our body. It helps our kidneys filter blood, flushes out the toxins, and ensures proper circulation in the body and flexibility of the blood vessels. Besides, our body is composed of 70 percent water. What does this mean to you? You need water to live! You should drink at least six to eight eight-ounce glasses per day.

Let's do the math. A gallon of water breaks down to sixty-four ounces, or two Big Gulp cups; two liters of bottled water; eight jelly glasses. The beauty benefits of water include supple hair and glowing, properly hydrated skin. Make the drinking experience sexy (or at least interesting) by buying a beautiful glass especially for your water or keeping a pitcher (think Waterford crystal, not Tupperware) of water replete with slices of citrus (orange, lemon, or lime) and your exquisite glass by your bed. Whatever you do, drink up!

Let's Get Physical

I am not going to insult anyone's intelligence here. We all know exercise is beneficial. Who among us hasn't sat on the couch with a candy bar in hand, watching Billy Blanks jab and kick his way into a new economic bracket? The experts agree that the best way to tackle weight loss is with a combination of cardiovascular exercises (five times a week) and weight training (three times a week).

Here are a number of things you can do right now without gizmos, gadgets, or a fancy trainer: *Walk, jog, jump rope, run up and down the stairs, work in the garden, dance, jog in place, clean the house, have sex.*

Sign up and move your moneymaker to raise funds for a variety of important causes. Help yourself by helping others. Here are five races that will engage the best of your Beautylicious self. (Check the websites to see if these races are in an area near you.)

Avon Walk for Breast Cancer; three-day walks; nationwide and globally; www.avonwalk.org

Revlon Run/Walk for Women; 5K run/walk supports women's cancers; New York, Los Angeles; www.revlonrunwalk.com

Walk to Cure Diabetes; nationwide and globally; www.jdrf.org

March of Dimes' Walk America; raises money to save babies from birth defects and prematurity; www.walkamerica.org

AIDS Walk New York; 10K walk; New York City; www.aidswalk.net

WORK IT OUT

Getting into tip-top shape is no easier for the Dolls than it is for the rest of us. Sure, they have trainers, but as Oprah pointed out, everyone still has to get on the floor and break a sweat. Here are some diet and exercise tips from a few fabulous frames:

Beyoncé hits the treadmill daily for at least thirty minutes and does 500 sit-ups a night. B's breakthrough? Accepting her body. "I don't want to be skinny. I like the fact that I look like a normal person."

Missy dropped the badunkadunkdunk in her trunk and then some by hitting the StairMaster for forty minutes and doing 300 sit-ups a day. She's banished pork from her menu, but

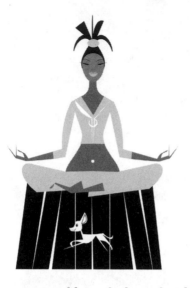

she still indulges in a few faves, only now she eats half a burger and a few fries instead of the whole thing. Ms. E's evolution: Measures progress by inches lost from her pants size. "The scale can be a bad thing. If you see you lost only one pound you feel like giving up."

Oprah got serious about weight-resistance training and alternates between upper and lower body work at least five times a week. She also does thirty minutes of aerobics each day, including jogging and power walking. The Great O's objection: a rigid diet. "I just eat smaller portions, and I still watch the refined carbohydrates. I favor fish, chicken, fruit, vegetables, and lots of soups. And I don't eat after 7:30 P.M."

FIVE VIDEOS THAT WILL MAKE YOU SWEAT

1. *Donna Richardson: Donna-Mite Aerobic Workout* and/or *Old School Dance Party*
2. *Billy Blanks: The Best of Tae-Bo Ultimate Abs* and/or *Ultimate Lower Body*
3. *The Goddess Workout with Dolphina—Bellydance for Fitness, Body, Mind, and Spirit*
4. *Pilates for Dummies*
5. *AM/PM Yoga for Beginners*

The Bod Squad

> *Start exercising your crucial areas earlier*
> *rather than later. The more you do before sixty,*
> *the more you can achieve at sixty.*
> —DIAHANN CARROLL

Stop, look, and listen to Pam, Diahann, and Eartha—foxiness is ageless. So, instead of fighting against what Mother Nature gave you, embrace it and enhance it through exercise. Here are the four basic shapes and tips on working with them:

Shape: Curves galore/hourglass
Babes who work it: Oprah, Tyra Banks, and Serena Williams
The look: Proportioned top and bottom, with a defined waist
Goal: Work your top and bottom with moderate weights
Minx moves: Running, walking, swimming, volleyball
Avoid: Heavy weight lifting and stair climbing

Shape: "*La guitara,*" Spanish euphemism for pear shape and
   big bottom
Babes who work it: Donna Summers, Mary J. Blige, and Eve
The look: Smaller shoulders, wide hips, and heavy legs
Goal: Tone and trim legs, thighs, and butt and build up
   shoulders
Minx moves: Swimming, walking, cycling long distances on
   flat surfaces, and low-intensity aerobics
Avoid: Stair climbing, step classes, and cycling up hills

Shape: Inverted pyramid
Babes who work it: Pam Grier, Vanessa Williams, and Queen
   Latifah

The look: Full upper body, rounded middle, and narrow hips

Goal: Tone upper body, trim waist, and build up legs and butt

Minx moves: Walking, step classes, crunches, arm curls, and cycling

Avoid: Swimming, rowing, exercises for the upper body that involve weights

Shape: Ruler

Babes who work it: Diahann Carroll, Michael Michelle, and Kelly Rowland

The look: Very slender, doesn't bulk up or add weight easily

Goal: To keep tone

Minx moves: Stationary bike, stair climber

Avoid: Everything's okay. Don't overdo it!

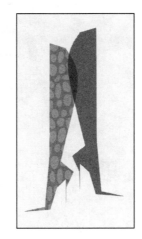

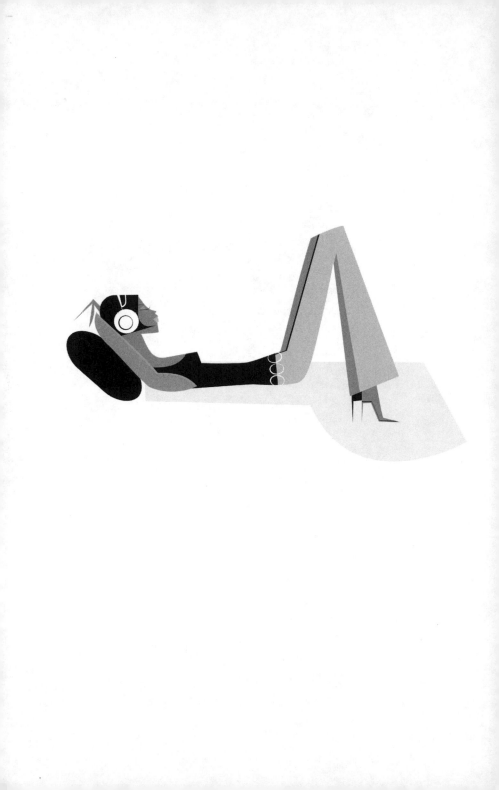

Chapter Three

Soul Power

*I wasn't born this way. One creates
oneself. I believe whatever I dream.
Whatever I dream, I want to do.*
—GRACE JONES

etting to know yourself, like building self-esteem, is a lifelong proposition. You know intellectually that you've got it going on and that you are one happenin' chick, but what about how you feel? Soul power is an all-access pass to the deepest parts of you in order to acknowledge your feelings unhampered and unimpeded. Nurture your spirit by being in constant communication with the Almighty, be it through prayer, chants, meditation, or just plain silence. Start your day and end it with a prayer of guidance and thanks. Your spirit also yearns for company, in the way of connectedness. Revel in the Almighty's presence. How? Enjoy and cultivate your connections with the rest of the world—family, friends, companionship with man's best friend, as well as the flora, the fauna, and the sun, moon, and stars! Cop a gratitude attitude. Say thanks daily, hourly, minutely for your blessings, no matter how big or small. Are you up and breathing? *Muchas gracias!* Understand spiritually, intellectually, and emotionally that you are made in the likeness of the Creator and that you are free. You are free to dream, to love, to create, to exhale, to feel pain and to move past it, to dance in poppy fields . . . you are free to be. And that alone may be the most subversive thing to tell a young black woman.

Me, Myself, and I

*I've always been the little kid on the outside of the
fence looking in at the greatness and all the things
you can achieve and have in the world. I've never closed
my eyes or my heart to what I could imagine or
what there is possibly out in the world. I think
when you close that off, you stop living.*

—PAM GRIER

Keep your eyes open, kiddo. You don't want to miss a thing. Always try to look at the world through your wide five-year-old eyes. That way you'll see the bloom on the rose or the flight of the bumblebee, which should serve to remind you that miracles happen every minute!

MY PHILOSOPHY

Socrates, Cornel West, and KRS-1 all have a philosophy, and, news flash, so do you. Yes, you have a philosophy—some guiding principles on how you're going to live, love, and leave the world a better place. Why not give yours some thought and jot it down. Written down, your philosophy gives you a glimpse of what you're all about and what your bigger goals are. Sure, you'll refine it a bit over the years, but you will always be clear on what guides you. Diana Ross's guiding belief is to "live my vision and to fulfill my purpose on earth, to learn to master life and to pursue happiness."

The tenets, according to Miss Ross, include:

1. Be true to yourself.
2. Help others.
3. Make each day your masterpiece.

4. Drink deeply from a good book.
5. Make friendship a fine art.
6. Give thanks for your blessings.
7. Pray for guidance every day.

You can keep your philosophy to yourself but it's even better when it's shared with a close, positive-thinking friend. Notice I said positive-thinking. You don't need Negative Nia telling you why your philosophy isn't worth the paper it's printed on or why it won't work in today's society. Hell, you don't need Negative Nia, but that's another story. A simpatica amiga will support you in striving to be the embodiment of your philosophy. With or without the friend, you have committed what you stand for and your guiding principles to paper, which is a powerful statement.

For example, one of my good friends is a personal assistant to a world-famous designer, yet she is never too busy or bogged down to jot down what her guiding thoughts are. She e-mailed me and said, "Life is too short, and each moment is what we make of it." So her personal rules became:

1. Do some type of creative project to release that part of my soul and to ease stress.
2. Always be in the middle of reading a book about positive thinking, or self-improvement, or any subject that fills my mind with what it needs to grow.
3. Mind my business. Literally! Focus on paying my bills on time and getting to work on time. On the job, focus on current projects and create new ones. And stay out of coworkers' affairs.
4. Wear pretty dresses and shoes, and carry bags. Feel feminine and lovely. I never know when I will meet my future boyfriend/husband.
5. Treat each person the way I would like to be treated.

Mine your dreams, examine what is important to you, determine what kind of person you would like to be, and write it down. Be bold, be confident, be honest, and you'll understand all that is beautiful within you.

ALONE IN MY SOLITUDE

Ever felt like the Brandy song, "Sittin' Up in My Room"? Of course you can relate to just sitting on your bed, staring at the walls wondering, "Is this all, Lord?" Trying to figure out what your mission in life is, hell, what your mission is right this minute. Feeling like the world is passing you by? It's cool—these are usually the times that the ideas come. It's quiet and you're contemplative. You put the questions out into the universe and you begin to get answers, maybe in a form you hadn't really noticed before: that big book on Egypt could spark the travel muse, or an illustration could remind you how you used to love to draw. Sittin'-up-in-my-room moments are priceless. Treasure them, for they actually are the wellspring of something great!

Living Single

Living alone doesn't mean you have to be lonely. Strike up a party for one in your little flat by indulging your wild and crazy side. Here are a few suggestions:

1. Whip up a batch of rum-soaked brownies and eat them for breakfast, lunch, and dinner.
2. Order those scandalous Marabou Slippers from Fredericks of Hollywood and practice your vamp walk.
3. Prop your feet up and have a marathon talk fest with a friend you haven't spoken to in a long time.
4. Read *Black Silk*, a book of black erotica, out loud.

5. Put your favorite posters up. *Sparkle* and *Love Jones* deserve a home.
6. Learn the Harlem Shake.
7. Rediscover the thrill of finger painting.
8. Watch cartoons. *Hey Monie* and *The Proud Family* are quite funny.
9. Wail along with Billie, Aretha, and Mary J.
10. Break out the china you bought at college or inherited and use it.
11. Dance the salsa . . . naked.
12. Revisit a pastime that you used to love but never seem to have time for—drawing, painting, knitting.
13. Read Baldwin and The Boondocks.
14. Veg out with an all-day beautylicious movie marathon. Stop the tape to learn or recite the lines that resonate with you.
15. Get a split of champagne and sip it with a straw during the above-mentioned marathon.
16. Write. It can be your autobiography, an ode to your beauty, a sonnet of love, or rhymes so raunchy Foxy Brown would blush.

The lesson: Live!

Inner Stoking

Spirit is the invisible force made visible in all life.
—MAYA ANGELOU

Cupcake, I know you're crazy busy and often stressed, as we all are, but one proven effective way to take it all down a notch is to center and renew yourself with the power of prayer. Carve out a bit

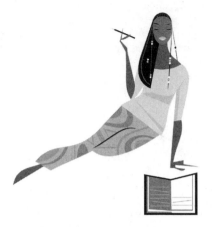

of space and get quiet. Matter of fact, pick a time each day—take fifteen minutes before you get your day started, or snatch fifteen for spiritual solitude as soon as you get in the house from work. Pray or meditate on all the good in your life. Thank the Creator. Visualize what you want for yourself and your loved ones. You might even want to create a spirit space, a little nook or cranny in your room that can be decorated with a few of your favorite things—plush silk pillows, the Bible, spiritual material for your journal, a pen, and a candle—to help you get into conversation with God.

MORNING GLORY

Sometimes the road may be rough and you may be weary, but you should try a little tenderness, with a song that moves you and gets you moving. For those days a shot of gospel in the morning can help you summon the strength to follow your own North Star. Although I thoroughly understand if "Pass the Courvoisier" is the only thing that will put that caboose in motion! Seriously, though, here are ten gospel faves guaranteed to get you to testify:

1. "Going Up Yonder": Tramaine Hawkins
2. "We Fall Down": Donnie McClurkin
3. "The Reason Why We Sing": Kirk Franklin
4. "Believe": Yolanda Adams
5. "Order My Steps": GMWA Women of Worship
6. "Let the Praise Begin": Fred Hammond

7. "The Potter's House": Tramaine Hawkins
8. "Open My Heart": Yolanda Adams
9. "The Battle Is the Lord's": Yolanda Adams
10. "Rejoice": Shirley Caesar

NATURE GIRL

Pam Grier takes to her horses and rides with abandon, and Eartha Kitt walks every day without fail in the woods with her dogs. While these fab icons have personas as hard-core city divas, they will all tell you it's their "country roots" that refuel them. Simply put, they always take time to commune with nature and to acknowledge its wondrousness.

One of the most powerful scenes in the television movie *Roots* is when Kunta Kinte's father raises baby Kunta up to the sky and says, "Behold the only thing greater than yourself." He was referring to the manifestations of a higher being—the twinkling stars, the full-of-possibilities moon, and the expanse of navy blue sky. There is a very primal connection between your spirit and nature; your soul longs for the stillness, universal wisdom, and the rhythms of Mother Nature. Your problems don't seem as big when you sit mesmerized by the perfect stillness of an azure lake. Look, if the Creator can create all that you see and control the wind, the rain, and the waves, it's a good bet that the Almighty's got your back. So go on, make a regular habit of strolling through the gardens, frolicking in the park, or daydreamin' by the pond. And say thank you for being able to be a part of all this magnificent beauty.

Music

The true test of a fabulous girl is not how many Jimmy Choos or Guccis she has in her closet but how many CDs and tapes she owns. You see, the Dolls love their music. It is part of their blood, it is their lifeline. It is no coincidence that most of the patron saints of beautyliciousness—Josephine, Eartha, Diana, Tina—are singers. Music is a religion. It speaks to the soul and resonates with the heart. It can be as simple as a haunting melody or a pulsating rhythm that transports you somewhere else.

The beautylicious babe loves to get lost in song, and she is the proud owner of an eclectic albeit sophisticated collection of musical stylings. She loves the bombastic sounds of Peter Tchaikovsky's 1812 Overture and Public Enemy's "Rebel Without a Pause," both of which get her adrenaline going. She knows no one can express a love jones better than Aretha with "Doctor Feel Good" or Patsy Cline with "Crazy." Whether she's from Harlem, USA, or Haarlem, the Netherlands, she's gone uptown with Duke Ellington's "Take the A Train," made a stop with Cassandra Wilson's "Take the Last Train to Clarksville," and seen the beauty of the stars through Frank Sinatra's "Fly Me to the Moon."

The beautylicious babe is a woman with a philosophy and a sound track, which makes her utterly delicious!

RIF, Baby!

Ms. Beautylicious lives for information. A believer in RIF (Reading Is Fundamental), she inhales every tome she can get her hot little hands on. Reading is a soul soother for her. She devours biographies and autobiographies, for she wants to know how other folks have handled the hills and valleys in their lives and all that it took for them to get to the mountaintop. She is a sucker for self-help books, and she always likes to check in with Iyanla and Dr. Phil to make sure she's getting it right. And, of course, she knows she can't call herself fab without a relationship with the fab lit gurus: Toni Morrison, Zora Neale Hurston, Alice Walker, Gloria Naylor, and Terry McMillan, or without a proper grounding in the classics, from Shakespeare to Ellison, and Proust to Mosley.

FIFTY BEAUTYLICIOUS BOOKS TO OWN

1. *Their Eyes Were Watching God* by Zora Neale Hurston
2. *Dorothy Dandridge* by Donald Bogle
3. *Brown Sugar* by Donald Bogle
4. *Confessions of a Sex Kitten* by Eartha Kitt
5. *Disappearing Acts* by Terry McMillan
6. *The Coldest Winter Ever* by Sister Souljah
7. *White Teeth* by Zadie Smith

8., 9., 10. *The Bluest Eye; Song of Solomon; Sula* by Toni Morrison

11. *Bulletproof Diva* by Lisa Jones
12. *In Search of Satisfaction* by J. California Cooper
13. *Cane* by Jean Toomer
14. *Buppies, B-Boys, Baps and Bohos* by Nelson George
15. *Miles Davis* by Quincy Troupe

16., 17. *The Women of Brewster Place; Linden Hills* by Gloria Naylor

18. *The Street* by Ann Petry
19. *Quicksand* by Nella Larsen
20. *Pimp* by Iceberg Slim
21. *Meridian* by Alice Walker
22. *The Boondocks: Because I Know You Don't Read the Newspaper* by Aaron McGruder
23. *A.L.T.: A Memoir* by André Leon Talley
24. *Basic Black: Home Training for Modern Times* by Karen Grigsby Bates and Karen Elyse Hudson

25. *The Hornes: An American Family* by Gail Horne Buckley
26. *Madame Bovary* by Gustave Flaubert
27. *Taste of Power: A Black Woman's Story* by Elaine Brown
28. *On Her Own Ground: The Life and Times of Madam C. J. Walker* by A'Lelia Bundles
29. *Race Matters* by Cornel West
30. *Wildseed* by Octavia Butler
31. *Invisible Man* by Ralph Ellison
32. *What Black People Should Do Now* by Ralph Wiley
33. *Black Girl in Paris* by Shay Youngblood
34. *Rock My Soul* by Bell Hooks
35. *DV* by Diana Vreeland and George Plimpton
36. *Secrets of a Sparrow* by Diana Ross
37. *Complete Stories of Dorothy Parker* by Dorothy Parker
38. *The Power of Style: The Women Who Defined the Art of Living Well* by Annette Tapert and Diana Edkins
39. *Jazz Cleopatra: Josephine Baker* by Phyllis Rose
40. *Quilting the Black-Eyed Pea: Poems and Not Quite Poems* by Nikki Giovanni
41. *Lady Sings the Blues* by Billie Holiday
42. *Always Wear Joy: My Mother Bold and Beautiful* by Susan Fales-Hill
43. *Why I Love Black Women* by Michael Eric Dyson
44. *Your Blues Ain't Like Mine* by Bebe Moore Campbell
45. *When Harlem Was in Vogue* by David Levering Lewis
46. The Bible
47. *I, Tina* by Tina Turner
48. *Drinking Coffee Elsewhere* by Z. Z. Packer
49. *I Put a Spell on You* by Nina Simone
50. *Gorilla, My Love* by Toni Cade Bambara

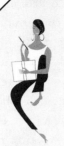

BEAUTYLICIOUS BELIEF: Create a space in your bedroom for uplifting books that you refer to in times happy and sad, books that you would recommend to friends in a heartbeat. While there is the Beautylicious Fifty, I keep the Uplift Six around me and read and reread Iyanla Vanzant, Neal Walsch, Marianne Williamson, Rev. T. D. Jakes, Rev. Bernice King, and Maya Angelou for comfort, clarification, and understanding. I found that when I was depressed or dejected, I would devour biographies and autobiographies. I would reach for someone I kind of liked or thought was interesting and I would be immersed. You'd be surprised how much I learned from Joan Rivers, Fran Drescher, and Maria Callas. Inevitably I finished the book feeling better and more optimistic. Why? It's when you start reading other people's life stories that you realize "no one gets a free ride in life." No matter how beautiful, talented, rich, etc., everyone has had setbacks, periods of no faith and unshakeable faith, and a bit of serendipity to get where they are. And that is the greatest inspiration to get out of bed and to exult in the business of living!

Lil' Bowwow

In many ways the dog turns out to be Ms. Beautylicious's best friend. And anyone can see why. Loyal canine is by her side as boyfriends come and go and fickle friends get dropped. Your pooch loves you no matter what. The dog is also an ideal pet because it is as sociable as you are. Mistress and pup take to the streets and everyone, including strangers, has something to say. FYI: Dogs are the perfect icebreaker, because while a man may not feel comfortable approaching you alone, a dog provides an easy conversation starter. And, doggone it, recent scientific reports have shown that owning a dog helps people live longer. According to numerous studies, pet owners have lower blood pressure, cholesterol levels, and stress. The canine is a friend, companion, protector, all rolled into a furry body. For single fab girls, owning a dog is a great experience in giving and receiving unconditional love, taking responsibility, and caring.

THE DOLLS AND THEIR DOGS

Eartha Kitt—two poodles
Pam Grier—German shepherd
Serena Williams—pit bull
Eve—Yorkshire terrier
Oprah Winfrey—nine doggies including the telegenic
   cocker spaniels and the oft-mentioned Labrador retriever
Janet Jackson—rottweiler

Always the showoff, Jo Baker had tons of pets, including several dogs, but her icebreaker was her pet leopard, Chiquita, with whom she would stroll down the Champs-Elysées.

Mis Amigas

The loneliest woman in the world is a woman
without a close woman friend.
—TONI MORRISON

In the words of the Divine Miss M., "Ya gotta have friends. The feeling is ohh so strong!" Ms. Beautylicious agrees totally with Bette Midler. She understands instinctively that she isn't an island and that a few pallies who are down for whatever and who have her back make life infinitely more livable, not to mention *mucho* fun. Your good gal pals are the ones you can call at some ridiculous hour of the night to cry about Brotherman, crow about a major accomplishment, or receive counsel on your dilemma of the moment. Studies have shown that your girls keep you healthy. According to the UCLA School of Medicine, people with a supportive social network are less likely to have high blood pressure, cholesterol, and blood sugar. And regular interaction with the gang slows the cognitive decline that may come with age. Best yet, your friends can help you find your soul mate. In a *Journal of Personality and Social Psychology* survey of seventy-four couples and their friends, the friends more accurately predicted the pairs with staying power than the couples themselves.

Understand that friendship can withstand long distances, periods of silence, and even major tiffs, but it can't withstand neglect. Friendship is like a big blooming flower; it must be tended to and cultivated. Yes, it can go a few days without water, but generally you must nurture it. Take time out to let your friends know that you love and appreciate them.

THE RULES OF FRIENDSHIP
1. Be flexible. Don't pout because someone didn't return your call within the hour.
2. Tell the truth.
3. Be forgiving.
4. Keep confidences.
5. Listen.

6. Be supportive.
7. Don't mix money, men, or Manolos, unless you're clear you don't want 'em back.

BOUNCE!

My friend Doris, who is affectionately (I swear!) known as the "Ole DB," offered this sage advice on friendship: "If the friendship does not bring you joy, end it." I forgot to mention that the Ole DB is quite blunt. However, in this case she's right. Not everybody who may be called a friend now is going to make it to the veranda with you in your twilight years. Why? There are the friends that you might have outgrown (the crew from high school) or grown away from (friends from the first job, the gym, or your old book club), because you and your interests have changed. Usually folks tend to let those friendships just fade away . . . with the answering machine, or with a compendium of excuses; it's a tad yucky, but everyone gets it. The joy-free relationships are a little more problematic in that you're trying to hang on to a "friendship" that really isn't there. Girlfriend is toxic. She may be a "Shlepprock"—you know, the Flintstone character; he was small, gray, mired in negativity and pessimism, and, in short, a drag. She may be supremely self-centered (let's talk about me!), and/or very righteous (I am right), or she betrayed your trust. Whatever it is, something deep within you always says no when she calls even while you're saying through gritted teeth, "Sure we can go . . ." Maybe you have been ignoring the pangs in your heart when you hear her voice. If you find yourself dreading phone calls, doing crossword puzzles while she's going on blow-by-blow about yet another injustice that's been done to her, do yourself a favor and let her go.

Cold? No. Sanity saver? Resounding yes.

At Your Service

Service is the rent you pay for room on this earth.
—SHIRLEY CHISOLM

What the first black congresswoman and the first woman to run for president meant is that you've got to give something back. Whatever it is you believe passionately in—the homeless, the environment, or the betterment of black people—support the cause with time, money, and a bit of elbow grease. Circumstances may not allow for all three, but any contribution is sorely needed and appreciated. Fight against AIDS or save the past-their-prime greyhounds. Find an outlet for all your concerns by browsing the Internet or checking a clearinghouse site like www.networkforgood.org. The beautylicious babe knows that she's been blessed with a bounty of talents and gifts and that volunteering, and giving a damn about her community and her people, are as natural to her as breathing.

THINGS TO DO

Get involved in the political process. Organize fund-raisers like Diahann Carroll, Lena Horne, and Star Jones do. How? Just look for the next race, be it for councilmember, alderperson, mayor, or president; identify the candidate you believe will best represent your interests, then volunteer to work on the campaign. It's also a great way to meet people!

Do your civic duty. Hey, get involved with your block association, tenants' association, or neighborhood association so that you can have an active say in what goes on around your cozy home.

Give a damn about your people. MTV and BET may suggest otherwise, but Dr. King's dream is still just that, a dream.

Continue the fight for equality by becoming active in either grassroots or established organizations. Bring some new life to your local branch of the National Association for the Advancement of Colored (I know—that's why it needs new life) People. Check out your local Urban League, too.

Support your alma mater. This is especially important to those who attended a historically black college. I know that you don't have the money to bestow millions on Spelman like fab icon Camille Cosby does, but you can send your school a yearly donation and have your employer match it. Or you can give time and energy like the fabulous Allen girls Debbie and Phylicia and the divine Jessye Norman do in the name of Howard University; simply join your local alumni chapter. Volunteer to do college re cruitment at high schools—anything to get potential students to your old college and foster goodwill for the college.

Find a cure. If you feel deeply about homelessness, pick up a hammer and check out Habitat for Humanity International Women Build, (912) 924–6935; www.habitat.org. Have you seen loved ones battle lupus, a devastating autoimmune disease that strikes black women disproportionately to other populations? Write a check to the Lupus Foundation of America and get more info from www.lupus.org.

Reach out and touch. What the world still needs is lots of love sweet love, and you have much to give! Dispense some hugs and kisses in the senior citizens' centers by reading and chatting with the elderly. Cuddle abandoned babies in the hospital or work with the drug-addicted. Walk and play with puppies and caress kitties at your local humane society.

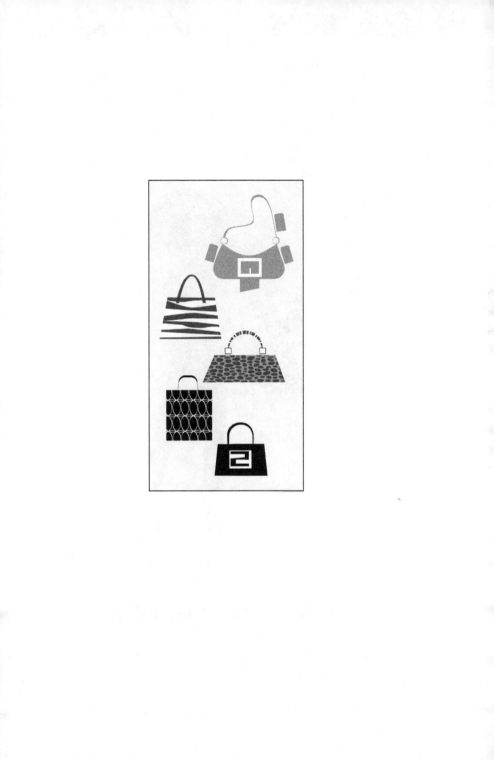

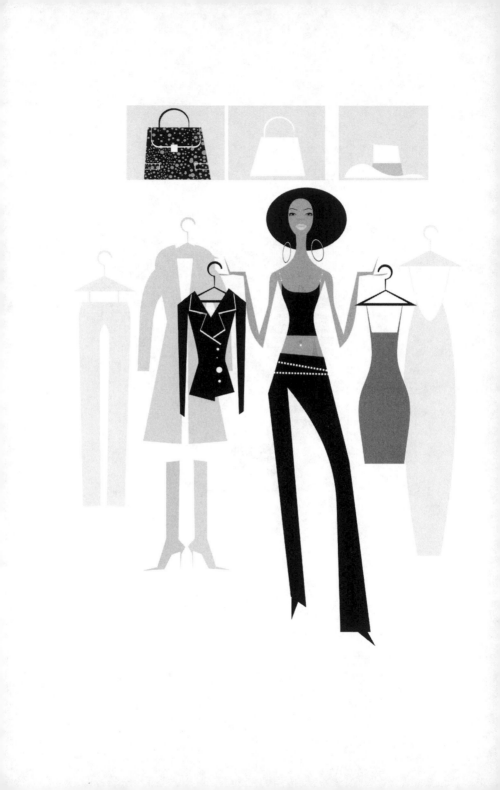

Chapter Four

Super Fly

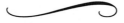

With hair, heels and attitude, honey,
I am through the roof.
—RUPAUL

obby Short said, "The difference between fashion and style is worth learning. Fashion is a follow-the-leader business, but style comes from you, how you see yourself . . . far beyond the reach of designers and magazine editors dictating what's 'in' this season or next." The dapper crooner is right on! Express yourself loudly and proudly. Yep, the beautylicious babe has an innate sense of style, but it is through trial and error that she homes in on her signature look. And she is not afraid to ask for help. Diahann had Josephine Premice show her a nifty bit of editing, and, what do you know, she's on the International Best Dressed List. In order to "work it" (the highest form of flattery in fab world) you have to truly revel in your clothes, dressing up any room that you sashay into. It's about taking your wildest ideas and desires and distilling them, narrowing down the looks into the best silhouettes and colors and utilizing your secret weapons—good undies and accessories. And, hey, not being afraid of looking crazy sometimes, until you get it right. Guess what? Once you find your style groove, you'll never howl, "I have nothing to wear!" again.

Build the Foundations

The most sensuous thing is when a woman has clothes on and you see some natural *body movement.*
—LOLA FALANA

Nothing kills a look faster than the wrong foundation garments or, worse yet, no foundations. True, the trussed-up boobies and booty is like so centuries ago, but just a glance on the street will tell you that most every *body* could use some support. Following are some tips on how to put a support system in place.

BUSTED

According to the bra experts, more than 70 percent of us are wearing the wrong bra. You know it's true, especially if you're still hanging on to the bra size you had in high school, even though you know you've put on at least ten pounds. What to do?

- ✦ *Get fitted.* Look for a trained fitter and have her measure you. You can find a fitter at any lingerie shop, or check your favorite department store for dates on their next fit clinic, in which fitters from the bra companies are on the premises.
- ✦ *Know what a good fit entails.* The straps around your body should be firm and comfortable. If the bra is too loose and rides up your back, you're wearing too big a back size (32, 34, 36). Wires at the front should lie against your rib cage and not rub, and your breasts should be enclosed in the cups. If you're bulging at the top (uniboob) or hanging out on the sides, the bra is too small. If the bra is gaping or wrinkling in the cup area, it's too big.
- ✦ *Get fitted every two years.* Or when you gain or lose ten pounds, whichever comes first.

Four bras that every girl should have, no matter what size she is:

Seamless is smooth and goes well under T-shirts and knits.
Convertible strapless accommodates all of your halters,
    bandeaux, and crisscross-strapped tops.

Sports keeps you from bouncing all over the place while exercising.

T-back/racerback works with sleeveless tops so straps won't show.

YOUR CUP RUNNETH OVER

The full busted (gosh, I love that euphemism) always look like they're having the time of their life in the movies and in the strip club, but one place that ain't so much fun for them is in the bra department, because there is a serious lack of sexy, cute bras. Here's the solution. Get your support on with the bras in the store. Your mams will love Wacoal (best minimizer), Bali, and Lilyette for their lifting and separating powers. Get your lacy, do-me bras online or by catalog. Check out Bravissimo, www.bravisimo.com, the UK-based shop that offers gorgeous bras in a variety of colors, swimwear, and tank tops and halters in cup sizes up to H. Also look to Bra Smyth, www.brasmyth.com, for a saucy assortment of Wacoal (they have a few hot numbers), Rigby and Peller, and lacy Lunaires in an assortment of styles up to H.

TA TAS ON TAPE

Trying to keep the girls high in a strapless or backless dress? Let's go to the tape: Take one or two strips of electrical tape and adhere it from armpit to armpit underneath your breasts like underwire for that pushed-up, overflowing look. A word of caution: This is really an A–B cup trick. C cups start to get . . . well, you know . . . sloppy, and over D, hey, floppy.

BOUND

No wardrobe is complete without a body shaper. Put the body shaper to work on days that you want to wear something figure hugging, and when you really only want to showcase the plush bottom and not the soft middle. This ain't your mother's girdle! No, today's shapewear is more comfortable yet still hardworking, thanks to spandex. What should you look for in selecting a body shaper? Give consideration to what you're trying to enhance, what needs to be smoothed down, and how much control you think you'll need to create the silhouette you desire. Please keep in mind, though, that this is not a miracle product—it cannot substitute for weight loss or liposuction, but it *can* enhance you.

Trying to whittle down the middle and banish bra bulge? Look to a slenderizing *body suit.* Tired of "it must be jelly 'cause jam don't shake" comments? Reach for a pair of *shorts*—what Ma used to call a panty girdle—a lightweight spandex affair that offers moderate-to-firm control. Depending on the degree of control, shorts can smooth and slim down the tummy, booty, and thighs, while keeping the dreaded jiggle in check. Approximate the sucked-in-gut look with a pair of *tummy toner briefs* for a more streamlined profile. And remember, to get the best fit you must try your shapewear on.

DECIPHERING THE CONTROL ISSUE

How do you know how much control you need? Literally and figuratively, let your gut be your guide:

> *Type of control:* Light, feels like control-top pantyhose.
> *Wear time:* All day.
> *Your gut says:* I am not at my fighting size. A bit paunchy due to water weight.
> *Occasion:* You're just trying to squeeze into tight jeans, skirt, or dress.

> *Type of control:* Medium/moderate shapewear with about 19 percent spandex. Generally will offer support panels for shaping.

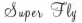

Wear time: All day.

Your gut says: This ain't water weight.

Occasion: You want the dress to hug every curve but the one between your bra and the waistband of your panties.

Type of control: Firm; can reduce your problem area by up to an inch. It has 18 to 25 percent spandex.

Wear time: About five hours a day.

Your gut says: I can't have someone ask if I am pregnant when I'm not!

Occasion: Shindigs that involve an ex-boyfriend or catty acquaintances you haven't seen in years, or any event that requires a camera.

Type of control: Maximum is the Fort Knox of shapewear; body parts are seriously secured. With a spandex count of 30 percent and either bones or panels, it puts excess flesh in check. Look to shave at least an inch and a half off your silhouette.

Wear time: Are we home yet? No longer than four hours, 'cause you will hurt somebody.

Your gut says: Sis, you gotta suck it up. Bring on the heavy-duty artillery.

Occasion: Anytime you're feeling like Orca.

Guerrilla Shopping

Hit the store with a take-no-prisoners attitude to get what you need and to enjoy the thrill of the hunt:

Have a purpose. Aimless was cute at sixteen when you spent the day in the mall in pursuit of boys and cheap entertainment. Today your time is more valuable.

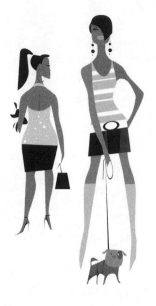

Know your wardrobe. Keep in mind the basic color scheme, the holes, the accessories, so if you do see a have-to-have-it item, you'll know right away that you have five of them already or that puce has no earthly place in your closet or next to your skin tone.

Make use of the salesperson. Contrary to popular belief, the salesperson is there to help you. Ask her about a piece you've been eyeing. Take it to the next level and ask how to hook it up. What does the manufacturer suggest? And then, most important, ask for her name and her card and let her know she did good. Create a relationship and soon you'll start hearing about the unadvertised sales and the little goodies that were saved just for you.

The biggest no-no. Never, ever abuse the salespeople. Sounds like a no-brainer, but you would be surprised at how many of your cousins go into the store and act as if they're auditioning for the role of Dominique Deveraux of *Dynasty*. Bag the condescension, the ordering around, and withering tones; all they say is that you're a rude creature with no home training. However, if the salesperson is the one grandstanding and acting like she can't be bothered to do her job, by all means fill the manager in on her antics.

FIND AND PATRONIZE BLACK DESIGNERS

Ms. Beautylicious knows the next step to true fabulousness is to not only know which designer's clothes work the best for her, but to know the designer. While Gucci is groovy, wouldn't it be even greater to find a neighborhood designer who could imbue

your wardrobe with a bit of soulful chic? Consider Erykah
Badu's loyalty to her designers, like Epperson and Cedella
Marley. "These clothes, they feel like they had you in mind
when they were being created," raves Erykah. And darling,
wouldn't it be fierce to become a muse to the next great designer? Think Audrey Hepburn and Givenchy, or Josephine
Premice and Givenchy, Catherine Deneuve and Yves Saint
Laurent, Diana Ross and Bob Mackie. Go out of your way and
off the beaten path to support a black designer, with dollars and
your feedback. You'll be sure to come away with a more individual look. Hit the black-owned boutiques and chat up the
owners. Get on their mailing list so that they can introduce you
to new finds and save the good stuff for you.

Just a few names to watch (these are the bigger names in the
business but they also represent the dizzying multiplicity of
black style and sensibility):

Stephen Burrows: Leader from the old school. He defined the
look of the seventies along with Halston. He's known for
slinky jersey pieces. Clients include Diana Ross and Iman.

Epperson: Known for his deconstructed dresses. Clients
include Erykah Badu.

Catch a Fire: Cedella Marley's (yes, Bob was her dad) line of
funky jeans, cords, and T-shirts. Clients include Eve and
Erykah Badu.

Eric Gaskin: Classic, elegant evening wear and fur. Clients
include Diahann Carroll and Lynn Whitfield.

Baby Phat: Kimora Lee Simmons's line of sexy urban wear
and great jean looks. Clients include Tyra Banks and the
hip-hop community.

Tracy Reese: Creator of flirty ladylike dresses. A fave with
fashion editors. Check out her lower-priced line, "Plenty,"
for fun, more casual looks.

Lafayette 148 New York: Edward Wilkerson's line of classic, tailored suits and career wear. Another must have for the publishing and jet-setting career women.

Sistahs Harlem New York: Models Carmen Webber and Shawna McDean teamed up with business wiz Carmia Marshall to create a line of edgy funkified tees and one-of-a-kind pieces. Clients include Jada Pinkett Smith, Jill Scott, and Iman.

MASS PLUS CLASS EQUALS SASS AND EXTRA CASH

Where is it written that style needs an unlimited cash flow? Target, H&M, Sears, Kohl's, and Wal-Mart should not be treated as bad words. These stores offer funky, trendy, as well as classic pieces at low prices. Use these stores to test-drive a trend, beef up your basic pieces, or give you more options for a saucy summer wardrobe.

Check out each store and utilize its strengths. For example, no one can do of-the-minute trends like Target and H&M. Pucci prints are the rage? Spice up your wardrobe with a bright Pucci-esque raincoat from these retailers for less than fifty dollars and wear it with aplomb. Sears, JCPenney, et al., are home to the basics. Pick up a few classic tailored shirts and cashmere turtlenecks from them. Mix and match with a few serviceable cotton or wool separates in your basic color palette to extend the life of your wardrobe. Espadrilles are the shoe of choice again; road-test the look courtesy of their shoe department. Why spend three hundred dollars only to rediscover that you weren't hepped up on that look the first go-round? Note: For the fuller figure, full busted, or the double-A girl, don't sleep on the Penney's or Sears catalog, which has a ton of foundation staples in a multitude of sizes. Wal-Mart and Kohl's do sportswear and workout clothes well. Stock up on shorts and sexy tees and weekend clothes from Old Navy. After all, you are getting the same silhouette you would get from its sister stores The Gap and Banana Republic for maybe a third of the cost. Go ahead, pair your bargain-basement finds with your designer duds with panache and put the dollars saved toward your "Saint-Tropez or bust" fund!

Necessary Accessories

While you may lose it with shoes and handbags, the smart minx learns how to care for million dollars in accessories she already owns as well as how to get her designer kicks and clutches for a few dollars less.

Handbag Savvy

A true aficionado never ever calls a bag a pocketbook. *Pocketbook* as a term is déclassé and passé. And a pocket book is what you read. A handbag, well, that's a bag. Now that you know what to call it, here are some guidelines for purchasing a good handbag. If you're going for a leather bag, look at the bag and make sure that there are no imperfections in the skin and that the color is even throughout. Do the same with vinyl and look closely for holes. Check the construction. Is the stitching even? Sloppy? Are there any hanging threads? Check the stress point—where the handles are attached to the bag—and make sure that the handles are secured properly.

Examine the lining of the bag to guard against puckers and ripples. Of course, handle the hardware—clasps, zippers, locks—and make sure that they're put on properly and, hell, that they work with ease. Leaning toward vintage? Make sure that the handle is secure, the frame is intact, and the fabric is of good quality. If the fabric is beaded, give it the once-over to be sure the beads aren't falling off. Lovely tapestry bags should be examined for moth holes.

HANDLE WITH CARE

+ When you're finished with a bag for the season, wrap it up in a pillowcase, towel, or sheet and put it away, to avoid scratches and nicks (this also includes canvas bags). That's why the designers give you a cotton drawstring pouch with your bag. It's meant to protect your purchase.
+ Stuff all bags with newspaper or plastic to keep the shape.
+ Clean your L.L. Bean bag or any canvas bag with a touch of Ivory Liquid. Of course, do a patch test in a small, discreet area first.
+ Remove the stains of rainy days and bouts of the dropsies with saddle soap.

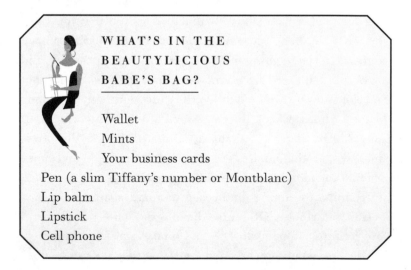

WHAT'S IN THE BEAUTYLICIOUS BABE'S BAG?

Wallet

Mints

Your business cards

Pen (a slim Tiffany's number or Montblanc)

Lip balm

Lipstick

Cell phone

Cute notepad
Palm Pilot
Comb
Compact (pressed powder)
Vitamins and/or aspirin in a cute tin
Keys
Tissues

Special assignations: Pull out the Vuitton Speedy satchel and fill with the above, plus:

Toothbrush
Clean panties
Condoms
Scarf
Hair essentials
Vial of perfume

Black-tie shindigs: Carry an evening clutch. The fab girl generally totes a lovely rectangular bag in Chinese brocade, sequins, or beads that match her dress, or in shades of silver, gold, ivory, or black satin. Inside she carries only:

Credit card
Twenty-dollar bill
Lipstick
Compact
Mints
ID, such as a driver's license
Cell phone

LOCO FOR LOGOS

Ms. Beautylicious is mad for designer bags. They are without a doubt the favorite accessory. We as a group have contributed mightily to the coffers of Fendi, Prada, Vuitton, Gucci, Dior, Chanel, and Coach. Here are a few observations on how to get the most out of your shopping experience and get the best bag:

Do not reward rude service. If you're in a shop or department store and the salespeople ignore you or are dismissive, don't buy a bag from them. I don't care if cash or an empty credit card is burning a hole in your wallet, do not stand for shenanigans just because you want the bag. Don't let anyone disrespect you behind the façade of exclusivity. You should get a hello and smiles from the moment you walk in the door, not to mention "May I help you?" No exceptions.

Keep all receipts and identification tags. These items will come in handy if you need to get the bag repaired. For example: Each Coach bag comes with a registration number. By registering you won't have to go through a lot of red tape or pay to get your bag fixed. Ditto, Prada's policy of providing a small credit card–size tag that includes the bag's name and quality assurance number. The card authenticates the bag so that you need not be in the ugly position of hearing the help whisper, "Er, this isn't one of our bags."

Be clear about the designer's return and repair policy. Who wants to think about repair or return after you've dropped a cool six hundred dollars on a bag? But the honest truth is in most cases, that money just bought you a fly bag, nothing more, nothing less. If you've noticed, the claims that the designer bag lasts forever and that it is worth every penny went out with the eight-track tape. The lone dissenter here is Coach. The company stands by the durability of the leather, craftsmanship, and construction, and for a $20 shipping and handling charge they are willing to fix any problem you may have. Prada is also pretty good about repairs, but they reserve the right to charge you if they feel the problem is your fault, as opposed to free when there may be a problem with design or material.

PRADA FOR NEARLY NADA

Aha! Gotcha. You're living for the designer bag of the season. You're willing to turn over the rent money. But it's time to understand the power of the media. If you're ready to sell your Ma for the latest (let's go there) expensive designer bag because, dang it, all the tastemakers, celebs, and socialites have it and *Vogue* tells you you need it, consider this: Celebs, editors, and that ilk get the bag for free, in exchange for being seen all around town with said hot item. There are ways around paying top dollar:

Trawl the consignment shops and eBay for gently used designer bags; they're usually less than half the retail cost.

Shop small towns. If you live in a big city like New York or Los Angeles, where designer bags are as necessary as oxygen, use your business trips to Butte, Montana to (A) find the Fendi you love and (B) purchase the Fendi you love at sale price, at any luxury retailer. Why is this so? Plain and simple, there isn't a run on these kinds of bags in the less stylish towns. Because of *Sex and the City*, MTV, and the five socialites that live there, the store is forced to stock a few Fendis, Pradas, Chanels, and Guccis. The only bag this trick doesn't work for is Louis Vuitton, which never goes on sale anywhere.

Hit the designer's outlet store. Sometimes the hit of the season may be in there in an offbeat color or just by dumb luck.

Get in the know and watch for sample sales. Of course, the hottest piece will be old news by then!

Travel abroad to outlet stores. There are Prada and Fendi outlets in Italy. Hit them with a vengeance. *Caveat:* This does not apply to the designer's boutique. You have to understand the dollar's value in Europe. Most of the time between the exchange rate and customs, it doesn't pay to buy Chanel, Dior, or Vuitton from their respective shops as there isn't much difference in price from the ones here, and you have to fight the Japanese tourists just to get into the store, for a limit of two or three bags. Why go through this extra schlepping? Except, of course, for the cachet of bringing home a bag from its motherland. In any case, why don't you spend the day at the garden in Versailles to fulfill your need for beauty and luxury?

Become friendly with the salesperson for your favorite bags. Once you buy something, exchange cards and let her know you want to be contacted about sales, trunk shows, etc. *Snob appeal:* In keeping with the shop's exclusive image, the salesperson will only solicit you as a preferred customer if you're a celeb with a stylist and posse in tow, or if you drop a lot of cash, and you do it frequently with the same salesperson. Still, it never hurts to ask.

Shoes, a Love Story

Okay, let's face it, you are a shoe whore, and I mean that in the very best sense of the word. You understand implicitly that a great pair of shoes can sharpen up a look. For example, Jimmy Choo stilettos can send an otherwise boring skirt-and-top look into the stratosphere. Your closet is overrun with every style and color of shoes, boots, slippers, and sneakers. You have never ever been able to walk past a shoe sale without trying something on. And, of course, there is the matter of the overdue student loan, because you had to have those supersexy Manolo mules. So you

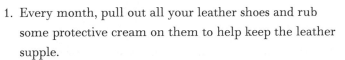

love shoes, but, honestly, what kind of condition is your collection of kicks in? Whether they're Christian Louboutin or Nine West, here are seven ways to save your soles:

1. Every month, pull out all your leather shoes and rub some protective cream on them to help keep the leather supple.
2. Don't store your shoes near a radiator or other heat source because they can dry up and shrink. Yikes!
3. Have rubber taps put on toes and heels, to protect soles from wearing so quickly.
4. Patent leather shoes can be cleaned with Windex.
5. If you're partial to suede, take your suede shoes to the shoe repair to be sprayed with a protective silicone coating, to prevent stains. Buy a suede brush and run it across the shoe or boot after each wear.
6. When your shoes get wet, stuff them with newspaper and let them dry naturally.
7. Polaroid shoes and staple the picture to the box. Rotate shoes seasonally, so that you don't have to wade through boxes to find the shoes appropriate for the current season.

Revival

This just in . . . nothing in fashion is ever new. The trends keep cycling around with the newness coming from either updated technology of fabric or an alteration of silhouette. One trend that you can always count on is the "Out of Africa" routine. Your spin? How about Ma's old dashiki worn as a tunic top, just slightly tailored to fit the body and paired with a pair of boot-cut jeans, or rock the dashiki gown by adding a slit on both sides for a sexy caftan, boho look. Another trend that keeps cycling around: back to the future. That's where the designers reinterpret the key looks of, hmm, let's say twenty years prior to the decade you're currently in. Beat the designers at their own game and figure out what the iconic references of that particular decade were. Get fresh with eighties wild style, that is, vestiges of hip-hop. Hit the trend quickly by accessorizing with door-knocker earrings, Kangol hat, or Adidas shell-toe sneakers. The only nod the original B-Girl can probably stand now is a sexy, fitted velour tracksuit. You get the idea.

EDIT

Elegance is refusal.
—DIANA VREELAND

Edit. This one simple word separates the fabulous doll from the ghetto fabulous girl. The fab doll knows to pare it down, be it accessories or head-to-toe designer outfits. Paring down is fabulous. Piling on? Ghetto (er, I mean urban, sorry, Sean) fabulous. Got it? Good! Before you leave the house, take one thing off. Before you leave your bedroom, consult the mirror and pick your point of focus. If it's going to be your incredible body that is being showcased to its best advantage in, let's say, a curve-skimming dress, why overpower the look and bore potential admirers by weighing yourself down with more gold and ice than the Cash Money Crew? And hey, while we're on the subject, if you're trying to look sexy, leave something to the imagination. In other words, keep your clothes on. Sure, serve up legs, but not legs, thighs, booty, and boobs. I know this is hard when all around you, wanna-be video gals have everything hanging out.

But just remember, the goal is to have someone say, "You look fabulous!" Not, "How much?"

CLOSET THERAPY

Why oh why is the prom dress with the garish neckline and un-flattering peach hue still hanging in your closet ten years after the fact? Is there any earthly reason you're still hanging on to the run-down Birkenstocks you bought during your boho stage in college? You get my drift. Clutter is not cool. Get rid of anything that you haven't worn in years ASAP. At the end of each season go back into the closet and make like John Gotti; get ruthless and methodical about your clothes purging. The sexy black dress that you used to work twenty pounds ago? Hello church clothing drive! The white blouse with the cigarette burn? Blouse meet Hefty garbage bag. You get the idea. Rule of thumb? If you haven't worn it in a year, trash it. If, however, you're sitting on a designer piece that is a little too of a particular moment, garment-bag it, send it to the back of the closet, and don't pull it out again until it's called *vintage*.

Fashion ID

> *I think clothes should convey a message, don't*
> *you? It doesn't matter if you're prosecuting a case, or*
> *interviewing someone on television, or running down*
> *to the corner store for eggs and milk, your clothes*
> *are the best billboard to your personality.*
> —STAR JONES

It's superficial, it ain't fair, but it's the truth: Clothes make the (wo)man. How you look says a lot about who you are. Although everybody's got different sides and different moods, it's the artful amalgamation of such that makes it something else. And that's fab style, the culmination of who you were, who you are, and who you want to be mixed with a bit of wit, insouciance, and a heap of soul. Now's the time to hone your style instincts. Stretch out on the bed with a pile of fashion mags and ask yourself a few questions: "What colors bring a smile to my face?" "What kinds of pants, tops, and skirts make me feel good and look good?" "What fabrics feel great?" "Whose wardrobe would I die to have?" Have some answers? Congratulations, you have begun the excavation for the glamour puss within.

MAKE A LOOK BOOK

Get in the habit of making a seasonal look book for yourself. A look book in fashion terms is a binder of photos of the designer's collection for a particular season. Create your own: Grab a binder, copy paper, tape, and some scissors, and at the beginning of each season cut out magazine and catalog pictures of the clothing and accessories that appeal to you. The look book is helpful on a few levels: It will reveal the common denominators—an untapped passion for strappy stilettos, turtleneck tops, or leopard prints—and it will offer suggestions on how to put a look together and help you add to your existing wardrobe.

HAVE FASHION ROLE MODELS

Ask yourself, what in your heart do you want to convey? And who exemplifies that look? Take a hint from Jennifer Lopez. She admires Rita Hayworth, Marilyn Monroe, and Jackie Kennedy. "Their look is classic, beautiful, sexy, and feminine all at once. I'm attracted to clothes that resemble that," gushed J Lo to Oprah. And with that she set out to create a modern, unique take on her faves, with the help of her stylist, of course. Branch out beyond Jackie O, Audrey Hepburn, Marilyn Monroe to find your style point of reference. Reach out to the Dolls for inspiration. Watch their movies. Go to the library and leaf through some old *Ebony*s and *Jet*s. Look at your parents' record album covers for looks that spark your spirit. Take notes: You will see

BEAUTYLICIOUS BELIEF: Say what you want about Jennifer Lopez, that chick brilliantly illustrates one of the most important tenets in playing dress up . . . confidence. Remember how she worked the Grammys in that diaphanous Versace gown with the V neck that plunged right to the honeypot? La Lopez never once tugged or pulled at the dress, or even looked the least bit shamefaced, all the while daring the men to look her straight in the eyes. While that doesn't qualify her for a Nobel Prize, it was quite impressive, because it was one of the purest manifestations of confidence. If you think I am overstating the case, look at the other girl singers who go for the no-clothes look on award shows. Folks are fiddling with their slit-to-the-eyeball dresses, giving off the bemused "My stylist thought this was a good idea" stare and looking generally uncomfortable. The lesson here is simple but powerful. *Remember:* Go daring, go crazy, go naked, but never go uncertain. Wear your clothes like you mean it, as an expression of your personality. Whether you're going for the haute call-girl look or just plain jeans and a tee, rock on like Jenny from the block and never look back, down, or sideways. Whoops! The important exception: Give yourself a major once-, twice-, thrice-over in the mirror before you leave the house.

that no one does pure couture, elegance, and classic looks like Lena Horne, Diahann Carroll, and Josephine Premice, and be aware that Michael Michelle is the new girl to watch.

Want to express your sexy, feminine side? Sidle up to Eartha Kitt, Dorothy Dandridge, and Lynn Whitfield, then understand that Halle Berry and Jada Pinkett Smith are the updates.

Interested in looks that are body-conscious, frankly sexy, and just this side of bodacious? Check seventies icons Lola Falana, Pam Grier, and Tina Turner, and know that Janet Jackson and Beyonce Knowles often fall into this camp.

If the iconoclastic, natural-woman look appeals to you, refer to Cicely Tyson, Abbey Lincoln, and Nina Simone for the proud Nubian queen thing, with Erykah Badu, India Arie, and Angie Stone ascending to the throne.

Want the whole world to pause when you walk into a room? Study the supreme-glam divas who work sequins, furs, fantasy, and *mucho* attitude. That's right, Jo Baker and Miss Ross created the category, Grace Jones took it to the edge, and now Naomi Campbell carries the torch for megawatt style.

Get in the habit of channeling your favorite Dolls for guidance when you hit the closet and use them as a jumping-off point for your own uniquely fabulous look.

DON'T GET CAUGHT OUT THERE

Being beautylicious is a twenty-four-hour job. You owe it to your public to serve up your special brand of glamour, even when you're walking the dog or running to the store for some milk. Besides, you don't want to run into Mr. Dream Man in some kind of crazy getup, right?

- ✦ Go through your casual clothes and get rid of the frumpy, shapeless stuff.
- ✦ Next time you buy a sweat suit, bypass Hanes and go more

upscale. Look to styles like low-rise, boot-cut track pants and fitted hooded jackets in luxe-feeling velour from Juicy Couture, Old Navy, The Gap, and Baby Phat. Or, if the dollars permit, upgrade to cashmere sweats from TSE. For the summer and warm climates, sexy shorts will suffice.

+ Matching hoodies work to cover up and ward off the night air. Keep the zipper at permanent half-mast.

+ Have a few colorful strappy tank tops or slightly snug T-shirts on hand to pair with your track pants or shorts.

+ Footwear can be anything from your basic sneakers to cutesy flip-flops.

Oscar-worthy Style

Ms. Beautylicious is always being invited somewhere, and sometimes she hits the jackpot with an invite to the shindig of all shindigs. That can be anything from the Oscars, the Grammys, the White House, the Soul Train Music Awards to a black-tie benefit. No matter, the breathless question is still the same: "Omigod! What will I wear?" A few tips:

Begin by taking a deep breath and uttering an affirmation like "I am beautiful and confident." Sounds dumb, but once you start hyperventilating about being in the same room with Halle or, heck, the exotic former Miss Guyana who doubles as the "witch in marketing," you're going to sabotage your confidence and your ability to enjoy the evening.

Which brings us to rule one: Make sure your confidence is on high. Rule two? Darling, be you, just turn it up another 180 degrees. Sling glamour. If you're into pants and comfort, look at evening suiting. How about putting your spin on YSL's "Le Smoking" suit, a tuxedo. Think about keeping it clean and spare in a sleek column of a dress with a hemline that works best for your gams. Take it up a notch by buying it in a luxe fabric. If you have a vision in mind and you have the time, call your tailor and collaborate on an outfit. Or you and the tailor or your trusted friend/stylist can customize a designer find (add flashy buttons, add a slit, etc.) to make it more you. Of course, the shoes should be high and very sexy and the bag should be very little and cute. If you're not wearing a suit, you should have a wrap on hand. Look for silky, fringy Gypsy wraps or classic silk wrappers. Yes, pashmina is yesterday's news, but it keeps you warm, so don't rule it out if it works with the outfit.

Now you're ready for the red carpet stroll!

HAVE A LIFESAVER

Nope, not the candy, but an outfit or two that you can jump into without a thought. Every season find one look that you rock when you can't think of anything else to put on, or for the last-minute invite. The beautylicious girl never says, "I don't have anything to wear."

Determine two lifesaver outfits. Make your picks from ensembles that you feel good in and have gotten feedback that you looked great in. If the low-rider Miss Sixty jeans and the halter top with the highest of heels always puts a smile on your face, well, Luv, you've identified your party-in-a-pinch outfit. And always have two LBDs (little black dresses) at your disposal. One should make you feel and look chic and elegant, and the other should have you feeling and looking hot like fire. *Comprende?*

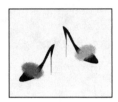

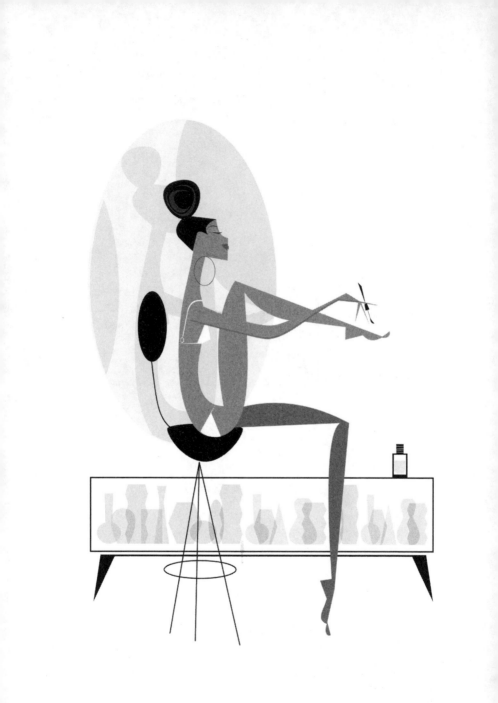

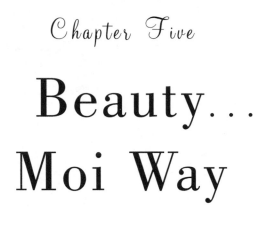

Chapter Five

Beauty...
Moi Way

When you're different, I think that's beautiful.
If you're operating on nothing but who you
are really, that always looks good.
—MACY GRAY

efine your own beauty. Don't leave that oh-so-important job up to the media, rap videos, the men you meet, your seventh-grade classmates, or even your parents. Rejoice in the fact that there is no $E=mc^2$ formula for beauty. Hey, look at Lena Horne and model Alek Wek, two very different looks, yet they're both iconic stunners. There is no pat formula; beauty just is. This is not to say that people don't try to define it for the rest of us. Scientists say it's in the big wide eyes and full lips because that's what made cavemen want to procreate. The "our kind of people" crowd still argue that light skin, an aquiline nose, and a slim build are the essential elements to be considered beautiful (oops, I forgot good hair); but these are frighteningly shallow definitions of a very personal and expansive word. Any of the dazzling Dolls past and present will tell you that while a few do max out in the pretty genes lotto, it's not always the artful arrangement of features that catapults one into true beauty. Nope, it's that Molotov cocktail mix of confidence, vitality, poise, and overall glamorization that wins the day and makes for the memories. Truth is, if we could figure out the $E=mc^2$-ness of beauty, what fun would it be? And how inclusive would it be? Ahh, so many questions, so little time. That's right, far too little time to waste figuring out how you stack up to the next dime piece. So, Cupcake, on the other side of the looking glass, beauty is really all about fun, play, and experimentation, because the Creator gave you all that you need. It's your inalienable right to bring the flourish!

I Am on the Top of the Mountain!

Such was the declaration my stylist friend continuously crowed the moment she was able to achieve the hair she always wanted coupled with a noticeable ten-pound weight loss. After years of wearing her hair in braids and schlumping down Seventh Avenue all covered up in padded coats, sweaters, and undies, Wally reinvented herself as a hot tamale with a mane of wild ringlets and a Coca-Cola–shaped bod. Now this metamorphosis sounds like it involved a little help from outside sources, but it didn't. Wally had the tools at her beck and call. It took a few years (you've got to factor in trial and error and your own stuck period). When she was mentally and emotionally ready for a new look, it was just about tweaking her hairstyle, exercising and fasting to shed pounds, and playing with a bit of makeup. Now she's always in the mirror smiling and saying, "Wally, you're one fine sister!" There is a message in Wally's madness for us all.

I must reemphasize that Wally's image change was really simple. She worked with what she had. She played around with different hairstyles, interrogated various hairstylists, dabbled with foundations to see which shade was best, decided that a weight loss was needed, and she went to work to attain her masterpiece. Once Wally was able to achieve the look she wanted, her perception of herself turned from merely lovely to Twenty-first Century Fox, and now girlfriend is leaving a lot of men with whiplash in her wake. The moral of the story? The top of the mountain is the only place for the beautylicious babe.

Glamorization

Look at yourself through the loving eyes of the three-year-old you. Channel the li'l muffin who loved to play with color, who was drawn to the fuchsia, aqua, citron, and burnt sienna crayons. Home in on the tot who was endlessly fascinated by her features—the roundness of her nose and the fullness of her lips and the difference of skin tones in her family. Let that little sweetie inform you on appreciating your outward appearance, and remind you of the joy of spontaneity.

Skin Tight

We've got a million delicious ways to describe our skin tones from café au lait to espresso, but the adjective that we really want is s-m-o-o-t-h.

OUT, OUT DAMN SPOT

Nothing is more of a drag than an acne flare-up. And for most of us, the zit can't come and go. No, it's got to leave its calling card, known as hyperpigmentation or just plain ole dark marks. Of course, one never knows when the next bump will come (er, usually for the big date or social event). Take a few preemptive strikes to keep pimples and the attendant dark spots down to a minimum.

ZAP A ZIT

6–12 Hours

Big greasy pimple staring you in the face in the A.M. and you have a date and a ticket to the Grammys in the P.M.? Hightail it over to your dermatologist ASAP for a cortisone injection. The doc will make an incision, drain the bump, then shoot it with cortisone to prevent inflammation.

The pimple should be on its way down before showtime. Not as flat as you'd like? Whip out your concealer (which should be one shade lighter than your foundation), apply to pimple, and blend, blend, blend. Follow with your foundation. Too much work? Use your dark brown lip pencil to go over the area and call it a beauty mark!

48 Hours

The bump that appeared on Monday needs to be gone by Wednesday. Reach for your standard-issue over-the-counter acne medicine, which contains benzoyl peroxide, and use it twice a day after thoroughly cleansing your face.

Whatever you do, don't continually douse your face with toner in the belief that you're diminishing the pimple. What you're really doing is setting off another problem in that the dry skin will kick up the oil production and then you'll have an overproduction of sebum, which leads to, yep, more acne.

DE-HYPE YOUR PIGMENTATION

Diminish dark spots before they start. Just get a pimple, burn, or an abrasion and you know you're prone to hyperpigmentation? Well, stop staring at it and begin applying hydrocortisone cream as soon as the bite, burn, or bump occurs. Wait for the pimple to flatten and the abrasion to close before applying the cream. Do this for five days. On the sixth, if there is a dark mark, apply a fade cream with 2 percent hydroquinone, and a mixture of alpha hydroxy acids like Black Opal Fade Cream, or one with kojic acids like Peter Thomas Roth's Lightening Gel, for up to four weeks.

GLISTEN UP

The poster girl for Le Jazz Hot, Miss Baker, believed in making her skin sparkle by showering herself in gold powder. Ageless bombshell Pam Grier, when asked how she pulls off not looking a day older than Coffy, said she uses good ole Vaseline, not on the camera lens but on herself for a vibrant shine. Take a tip from two proven showstoppers: Glowing, touch-me-please skin is a must. You can create your own glow by updating the Dolls' tricks: Crush up that old gold, bronze, or copper powdered eye shadow or bronzing powder and mix it into your baby oil. Apply all over for a sensual sheen.

CONCEALED!

This just in: Sporting full-face drag to work out, walk the pooch, or to scale Mount Kilimanjaro is just that, a drag. C'mon, at best it telegraphs high maintenance. And at its worst: "Yikes, that girl's got something to hide." You can, however, run a few laps or meander at the dog run and still give good face. Rock these undetectable tricks for the "Me, only better" look: Well-defined brows set the pace for the face. Concealer (a dab will do ya) in a shade close to your skin tone, to cover dark spots and dark circles under the eyes. A coat of waterproof mascara (activity = sweat) to open up those brown orbs, and a slick of a soft, muted lip gloss.

The Flirty Glance

A few eye-spy looks to try:

> *Bambi:* Janet (Miss Jackson to you) takes the doe eyes to the
> max with the help of false eyelashes. Cut a strip of lashes

into small sections, pick each up with tweezers, and apply a strip of glue to the back of lashes. Apply the shortest where your own lashes are shortest, longest at the center. Want to take it to Bambi Does Dallas? Simply add the longest lashes to the corner of the lower lid à la Lola Falana. Apply two coats of mascara once lashes are on. Follow with a clamp of the eyelash curler.

Crystal vision: Shade your eyes with a nude-color base. Apply a touch of eyelash glue to several Swarovski crystals and affix to the lid for an Alicia Keys sparkling-ingenue moment.

Kohl mine: Mary J. and the above-mentioned Alicia Keys work the updated Nefertiti liner look. Use a kohl liner, rim the eyes, and smudge out the outer edge of the eyes with a sponge-tip applicator.

Smoke alert: Everything isn't in shades of black or gray. You can have smoky eyes with any shadow. The softest take? Opt for a chocolate powder shadow, apply it over the entire lid, and lightly rim the bottom of the eye. Follow with a light dusting of white pearlized shadow—pat it on the inner lid (toward the bridge of the nose) then start blending out toward the outer lid. Line eye. Luminize brow bone with a very light gold shadow.

Faux faux lashes: Predust lashes with baby powder and add a couple of coats of thickening mascara.

The Young and the Restless

Party girl extraordinaire, you never leave a shindig until the chairs are being put up and the last bottle of Moët has been swilled. Of course, that lifestyle leads you to fire, brimstone, and, ahem, puffy peepers. You can soothe your lids by lying in bed for a good part of the day with cucumber slices or chamomile tea bags on your eyes, but who's got that kind of time? After all, you've got work to go to, and you are an hour and a half away from late. What to do? Go the Sade route. The sexy crooner manages to pull off one of the chicest looks in the most low-maintenance way. She keeps the mystery going by being a woman of few words. Hey, that can work if you're just pulling yourself out of bed.

Your brand of smooth operating: Apply a dollop of pomade. Brush hair back and smooth it into a low-slung ponytail or braid. (Short hair Dolls, simply gel and brush hair back.) Brush brows and shellac lips with an "I'm alive" red lipstick. Button your white shirt over black boot-cut or cigarette-leg slacks. Reach for the gold hoop earrings, the bigger the better. Fly out the door with perfume on high and voice low and sultry.

What You Need in Life

You've already got money, power, and respect. But what are the five essential beauty items no fab doll would be caught without?

1. *A signature lipstick shade.* You probably have five thousand tubes strewn around the bedroom, but which shade is the one that makes you feel as if you can conquer the world? What shade always garners, "Wow, I love that color on you"? Ten to one it's the same shade. Make sure you always have a tube on hand. Also on the vanity, a red lipstick that says sophistication, fun, laughs, and good time, and a sexy nude shade that goes from chic simple to *vroom* sexy with the wave of your shimmer gloss wand. *Fab for life:* They've discontinued your fave Groovy Grape and you didn't get the memo? Have

your lipstick duplicated and kept on file at Three
Custom Color, www.threecustom.com.

2. *A red lipstick.* Red will always signal passion, danger, and
   sex. Keep a shade of rouge in your beauty arsenal for your
   own signaling. How to find the red that's hot on you? Play
   with a few. Buy the one that makes you feel as glamorous
   and as beautiful as Halle Berry on Oscar night. *Fab for life:*
   Let him know that your middle name is still Danger by
   applying a hint of shimmer gloss in the middle of the
   lower lip.

3. *A great base.* Notice I said *great. Great* means the shade
   matches your skin exactly. Make the best match by
   swatching your jaw line with foundation and then
   stepping out into the sunlight with your mirror to see if
   the color matches your skin tone. When you find the
   foundation that totally matches—still a tough proposition
   for us—you've got to buy by the case. Six brands that
   really run the gamut for our skin tones: Black Opal, Iman,
   I-Iman, Fashion Fair, MAC, and Estée Lauder. *Fab for life:*
   Get your foundation custom-made by Prescriptives (at
   most department stores).

4. *Fragrance.* Find a scent that makes you feel sexy, brave, and
   upbeat and let the world in for a whiff! *Fab for life:* Stack
   up your pennies and splurge for a customized scent.
   Introduce yourself to the perfumer of royalty and the
   terminally chic, Creed. The venerable French perfume
   house, with assistance from you, will create an individual
   scent, housed in a leather atomizer, for $300 to $1,000 for
   1.7 ounces.

5. *Sunscreen.* Good black won't crack, but it will burn. *Fab for
   life:* Reach for a sunscreen with an SPF of 30. While the
   label hussies will go in for Clarins, don't overlook Neutro-
   gena and Avon for state-of-the art soothing sunscreens.

Insider Intelligence

Understand one thing: The cosmetics industry is a business built largely on emotions, aspirations, and dreams. So don't always fall for the hype that the more expensive or designer skin care or lipstick is always better. What is better is the marketing and advertising budget as opposed to the drugstore or door-to-door brands. Do not sleep on such brands as Avon, Revlon, and Mary Kay, for they have pioneered many of the industry's biggest innovations, like the use of alpha hydroxy acids in skin care or lip liner/gloss pencil and they have the technology. The beautylicious beauty maven knows that those expensive hundred-dollar-an-ounce creams are cute, but the real buys come from following these simple tips: (1) Always cruise the Avon brochure. Avon turns out state-of-the-art skin care. (2) Maybelline, CoverGirl, L'Oréal, and Revlon are always trying to outdo one another in making long-lasting products and making pretty colors for both eyes and lips. Maybelline's Great Lash is still the leader in mascara, and Revlon and CoverGirl have perfected the long-lasting lipstick. (3) Short on funds? Splurge on the luxury item if it's a product that will be seen in public; that is, you should always have at least one lipstick housed in a sophisticated black lacquer case, ditto for the face powder. One caveat: Never skimp on foundation for your skin. Buy the best.

Camera Fly

What can you do to make that Kodak moment one you'll treasure? Look slimmer by holding your shoulders down and slightly back, for an elegant swan-neck look. Or turn your body forty-five degrees away from the camera and turn your shoulder and

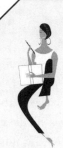

BEAUTYLICIOUS BELIEF: First day away at college, and the line for student ID photos was very long. What was the holdup? I found out later on that night. It seems my roommate, Natalie, took at least a half-dozen photos until she got the right one. May I say it was a beaut; a three-quarter head shot with emphasis on fabulously kohl-rimmed eyes and pouty lips. The ID picture was a vision straight outta *Elle*. Hence, the photographer's willingness to entertain Natalie's tomfoolery. Everyone else's ID photo looked like the startled deer in the headlights. How did she do it? "I know my best angle," she sniffed. "Oh," was all I managed to choke out. Okay, what sounded like a clear case of vanity and an idle mind back in the day is actually the first tenet of taking a photo you'll love.

BEAUTYLICIOUS TIDBIT: Gather up your best buddy, the Polaroid camera, and a couple of packs of film and shoot away! Try different angles and expressions. Go over the photos to find out what you like. Most important, think good, positive thoughts. The eyes never lie.

head to face the camera. Slim down flabby arms by slightly bending them and holding them away from your body. If you are in a group picture, place your arm around someone's waist.

Afraid that your so-called facial flaws will magnify to the size of Texas? Downplay the feature you haven't come to terms with by the way you hold your head. Mariah Carey was merciless about the three-quarter angle shot from the left side, head tilted slightly downward so that her nose would appear slimmer.

Utilize advance warning from the resident clicker. Hit the bathroom and add a bit more makeup, especially another layer of mascara for an open-eye look. Keep blotting paper on hand to soak up the oil and then follow with a dusting of powder for a cleaner, smoother look.

$\mathcal{N}$ude $\mathcal{A}$mbitions

Baby, bare your wares with wild abandon. Strut, preen, sashay, and parade what your mama gave you. Caress those curves, embrace your build, stroke your skin. You sing the body electric, because that's what it is. Good vibes and positive currents run through those who can see the magic of their bodies, love handles and all. Loving and accepting your body *unconditionally* is a wondrous thing. It just feels good. It also frees up precious brain space for concerns like how to achieve world peace, instead of visions of Porky Pig running through your head. However, if you're thinking, "That's Petunia, to you," know that you can obtain beautylicious babe-in-the-buff status and a better attitude. Just think like a bunny, a Playboy bunny, that is. Beautylicious buds and bods *Playboy* Playmate Nicole Naraine (Miss January 2002) and 1990 Playmate of the Year, Renee Tennison, share their secrets on how to showcase your body like the work of art that it is:

- *Get comfortable with yourself.* How do you get there? Again, a lot of face time with the mirror. Look at your body. Okay, now let's look at it lovingly. I know the first glance went right to the stomach pouch or the so-called cottage cheese thighs. Flip the negative script and start appraising everything positively.
- *While you're in the mirror, learn what makes you sexy.* If you think your butt is one of your best assets, play around

and come up with some poses that you think highlight you. Fresh out of ideas? Look at a *Playboy* magazine or some of the old cheesecake shots from *Jet.* There is no shame to your game. Have fun!

💗 *Adjust your mind-set.* Whatever the situation, know what you're going for. New rendezvous? Heck, the introduction of the Polaroid camera. Think, "Hell, I am hotter than July and Miss July." The bonus? You'll act on the thought! Get hip to what Miss July, Ma, and Dr. Phil already know. It's all about perception. Remember, "If you think you're the bomb, then you're the bomb!" Sign off from your mirror time with that loud declaration.

💗 *Quit comparing yourself to other women.* Know what makes you special. The competition isn't between you and his last girlfriend, the random hoochies, or J Lo; Sis, you are your only competition. Look inward to find out what's great about you and know that, again, it's not about perfection. The Dolls we've been talking about aren't perfect. Of course, feel free to up your game by making a commitment to care for your body in ways that will make you feel sexy and strong. Try yoga, tai chi, or belly dancing, which all offer residual benefits, aside from strength and a little weight loss!

The bottom line: Strip yourself of tired self-perceptions and you'll be ready to take it off for yourself, your man, or (dare I say) the camera.

The Hair Down There

THE WELL-GROOMED THATCH

You know the deal with waxing; the aesthetician has you splayed out like a chicken and pours a bit of warm wax on a portion of your private parts; then she lays a bit of cheesecloth on the wax and snatches it up, one millisecond before your brain registers *scream!* If waxing is a pain, take two aspirin before you're waxed to dull the pain. Also, after waxing don't go out in the sun for twenty-four hours. Wax a couple of days before the beach. Is bald for you? Because our hair is curly, do-it-yourself shaving and cutting is likely to produce ingrown hairs and truly unsightly razor bumps. Did I mention the pain? With that thought in mind, understand that the bald coochie is more problems than it's worth, unless it's a requirement of your profession (I won't go there!) or your desire. Why is this even up for discussion? We're a culture that doesn't like hair, except when it's abundant on our head, and we're also part of a culture that's not big on natural odors and sweat, which pubic hair holds. All that talk about Brazilian waxes bore you? Keep your little thatch intact and make it sexier by sprinkling a tiny bit of essential oil or a bath oil blend downtown.

COLOR FORMS

A few adventurous cookies want the mane and muff to match, or they may be plain tired of plucking gray hairs. What to do? Well the first line of action is to inquire at a salon that does bikini waxes if they would do color as well. If so, just remember that pubic hair is darker and in order to get an exact match you need to get a shade lighter than your hair color. Going for a blond on bronze effect down below at home? (Hey, we don't pass judgment!) Reach for a bleach made specifically for facial hair. This is a delicate undertaking, so make sure you avoid getting bleach in the vaginal lining. To be on the doubly safe side, just color your pubic mound and not the hair on your labia. Further protect yourself by coating the labia with Vaseline and covering it with tissues. Apply bleach or dye with a cotton swab or a clean mascara wand. Comb through first in the direction of the hair growth and then the other way. Don't leave the bleach on for more than twenty minutes or it could irritate your skin. Finally, wipe off any excess product before jumping into the shower. Omigosh, you spilled the bleach? Don't panic. Rinse yourself thoroughly with water. Soap will only increase the irritation. If the area starts to burn, try applying an over-the-counter hydro-cortisone ointment such as Cortaid.

Naked Attitude

If you've got a body, flaunt it. I'm a
body-conscious girl. I say why not show the
guys what sex appeal is all about.
—VIVICA A. FOX

Okay, you and your booty are the best of friends now. Listen to Ms. Sly Fox and take your act on the road, with a few shame-lessly indulgent treats and tips from the grad course of body appreciation:

- ❤ Spend a few minutes padding around your abode in your birthday suit. It gives your body a chance to breathe, and you get the joy of feeling totally unencumbered. Don't forget to close the blinds so that the neighbors don't get a free show!

- ❤ Slip into a rose milk bath. Try this sexy update to the classic milk bath, Diahann Carroll's favorite soak: Add a quart of milk (or the equivalent of powdered milk) to warm, bath-temperature water and swirl it around. Add a few drops of sesame oil, to soothe dry skin. Or take the milk bath to the next level by adding ten drops of rose essential oil (look to the health food store or the Muslim brothers on the corner) and sprinkle a few handfuls of rose petals into the water. Engage your senses! Revel in the lush visuals of the floating petals, soak in the soothing and conditioning powers of milk, and inhale the sultry sweetness of the rose. Be in the moment and enjoy how the bath flirts with your sense of touch, sight, and smell. Heighten the experience with a glass of champagne and a languid jazz track playing in the background.

❤ After you bathe, instead of doing the once-across with the towel to dry, go lie underneath a ceiling fan or a slightly opened window. Again, about those neighbors . . .

❤ Caress yourself with a mega-rich, opulently scented body cream. Smooth it on from your neck to your feet very slowly, and get reintroduced to the feel of your skin. The best whiffs for sensual healing are the orientals, which refer to the various notes of the fragrance and are reminiscent of the Far East, with such exotic ingredients as cinnabar and amber. In other words, the old school scents like Yves Saint Laurent's Opium, Chanel's Coco, or Calvin Klein's Obsession are supremely sexy as body creams. Want subtly glistening skin and a boudoir-right tuberose scent? Reach for Michael by Michael Kors.

❤ Swathe your body in nature's fibers. Slip into a next-to-nothing silk chemise from La Perla or Miss Vicky's, or into Swiss cotton thongs from Hanro. Slide under 300-thread-count Egyptian cotton sheets (more on that in chapter 10).

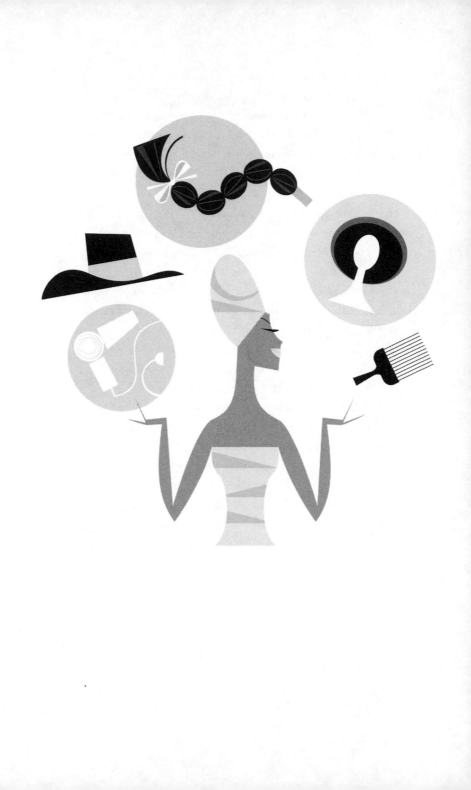

Chapter Six

Mane Intrigue

I want the great masses of people to take
greater pride in their appearance and to
give their hair the proper attention.
—MADAM C. J. WALKER

air is the beautylicious babe's obsession. Yeah, it also happens to be the obsession of women in general, but hey, I am not talking to them! We put so many demands on our poor follicles. Listen to yourself: The hair's got to shine, be perfectly sleek or perfectly curly, be gloriously long or seductively short, and it's got to be the envy of sisters within a hundred-mile radius. It's a wonder the poor strands don't fall out because of expectations exhaustion! And we're not even going to get into the creative ways we express ourselves through our mane. A quick glance at the Dolls' pantheon of 'do one-upmanship reveals stunts like singer Joyce Bryant pouring silver radiator paint on her hair to go one better than La Baker and emerging as the "black Marilyn Monroe," and Patti LaBelle sporting strands freeze-sprayed into fans. Grace Jones's fierce declaration of strength and beauty in her sculpted high-top fade. And Erykah Badu's and India. Arie's ultimate act of defiance: They shaved off their hair to free themselves of the sway hair holds over black women. Spectacular hair begins, as the Great Madam Walker says, with proper attention, also known as love.

The road to a marvelous mane begins when you make peace with your hair. Shoot positive vibes of love and appreciation right through each strand. In other words, create a relationship with your hair. Then when you and your hair start to go steady, locate a part-time lover who can partner with you to make your hair look its best. It's also time for a few tricks to keep the mane

fresh even in the toughest of situations be it the morning after—
you can glide out of his bed without looking like Buckwheat—
the global trot, and when you're just flat-out broke. Marry the
elements of attentiveness, a proper hair-care regimen, and an ac-
knowledgment of your lifestyle, and voilà you've got hair that
offers versatility, freedom, and excitement, or fab hair. Celebrate
and nurture your mane. Madam Walker would be proud.

Team Me Revisited

> *There will always be a need for*
> *the Negro beautician.*
> —ROSE MORGAN

The hairstylist is the linchpin of this whole operation, because
we all know that if the hair doesn't look good, the beautylicious
babe just isn't feeling good.

HOW TO FIND THE TEAM LEADER, AKA THE HAIRSTYLIST

Take a poll. Ask anybody—friend, foe, stranger, or family member—whose hair you admire for the name of her stylist and the
salon.

Peruse the hair magazines. Take note of the styles that you
like and the stylist credit. Go to the salon and have a chat with
the stylist.

Chat up potential stylists. Schedule a few get-to-know-you
consultations. This will give the stylist the opportunity to examine your hair, ask questions about what you want and your
hair history, and tell you what is achievable. The consultation
should also give you time to check out the stylist's personality—
pleasant, dominating, know-it-all, just plain bitchy—his or her

specialties, recommended products, and whether the stylist's method of hair care is in sync with what you want. Just like when you have your first date, Brother will always tell you what he doesn't want to do, so will your stylist. If you want a roller set and he talks about the greatness of a blow out, or repeatedly tells you that he loves relaxed hair but not natural, move it along and go to another stylist.

Take in the general ambience of the salon. Unfortunately, with a black salon you're going to be there awhile so you might as well make sure you're comfortable with the place. Note the level of professionalism of the stylist and of the salon overall. Don't accept a salon that overbooks, goes in for loud and wrong gossip, or acts as an outpost for the Homeboys Shopping Network.

Get real! Once you have told the stylist what you want, be prepared to hear what actually can be done for your hair. If he is telling you that your hair is damaged and that a few inches have to go, respect his professional advice. Remember, healthy hair should be your foremost goal.

Confess to tress mess. Be up front about your hair mishaps— the Copa you put in it five months ago, whether you are taking medications, and if you know from trial and error that a regular relaxer is too much for your soft hair.

Be up front about how much work you are willing to put in. There is no use getting an elaborate hairstyle if you have no interest in maintaining it. If you don't have the time, let's say, to curl your hair at night or go through some elaborate process in the morning, please tell your stylist so that he can create a minimal, easy look for you.

Be on time. Call if you're going to be late.

COME AND TALK TO ME

Everyone has a hairstyle horror story. Who among us has not suffered through the "I said trim but the stylist heard cut . . . a lot" scenario? Or you wanted to be a golden blonde, but you left in shades of scary spice? Going to the hair salon should not be a frustrating experience. The key to avoiding hair hell? Communication with your stylist. Some tips on how to communicate effectively with your stylist, so that you're not "distressed":

✦ *Get dolled up, especially if this is your first time with the stylist.* Your stylist needs to get an idea of your entire look. Your personality, body type, face, and wardrobe are as important as your hair type in deciding your ideal cut and color.

✦ *Bring in photos of the hair color or the haircut you want.* When you show the stylist specifically what you want, she will be able to take the idea and tailor it for you.

✦ *Ask your stylist for his or her definition of a trim.* Yes, we want to hang on to every inch of our chemically/ environmentally challenged strands, but we can't. However, before the stylist goes for the shears, he or she should show you in the mirror how much needs to be cut and explain why. When you are absolutely clear and cool about it, give the okay.

✦ *Show some appreciation!* Good communication is a two-way street. If your 'do turns out to be "da bomb" say so. If you love what the stylist did, send a thank-you card. Not only does that make the stylist feel good, but a little positive reinforcement goes a long way.

FROM THE EX-MANE MASTER TO THE NEXT

Your stylist just isn't cutting it. You're not excited about your hair, he is just personally intolerable, or you really want to go somewhere else to get your hair done. Whatever the reason, you don't have to slink away from your stylist like a thief in the night or walk through back alleys to avoid him. Try a little honesty and tell the stylist that you are not happy and you would like to try someone new. Now, if you really like your stylist, you can add a little more, such as, "I love your classic styles, but I am looking to go in a funkier direction. . . ." If the kindest words you can muster are "You and your work sucks," well, keep the speech to adios!

HOW TO FIND A 'DO FOR YOU

The first step is to determine what you want your look to be. Figure out through style inspirations and pictures what you want your primary hairstyle to look like. Make sure you opt for a style that flatters your face above all else. Sounds like a *duh*, but think of how many women are walking around looking like a Shih Tzu because they wanted long locks, yet the hair overpowers their small face. To make life easier for you, note that there are really only six basic hairstyles for us. The rest is just a riff on a theme. The six 'dos can be found in any issue of *Ebony* in any decade. They are

The Afro

At its peak: A perfect orb on top of your head; had to be the seventies.

Update: The textured piecey free 'fro.

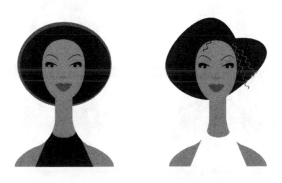

The Pageboy

At its peak: College. The style of choice for every college girl with shoulder-length hair and for those who haven't had a hair change since college.

Update: The basic bob is now cut into longer layers for sexiness and movement.

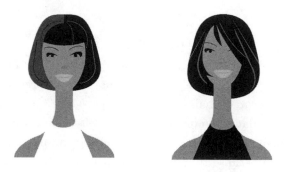

Braids

At its peak: Sixth grade; when Mom didn't feel like being bothered with you or your hair she would put in plaits or skinny cornrows.

Update: Revisit cornrows via the sexy way Janet Jackson wore them in *Poetic Justice*. Do the twists and consider locks.

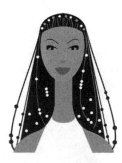 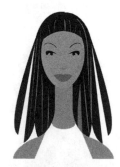

The Slicked-back 'Do

At its peak: High school. The short hairdo was always
greased and brushed within an inch of its life. Either you
were giving up Jo Baker or the local bully. There was no in
between.

Update: Texturized to highlight the natural curl pattern.

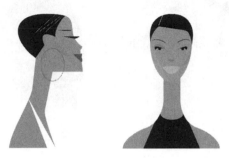

Long Hair

At its peak: Freshman year of high school. When not bound
in a ponytail or braid, hair cascaded down your back with a
tight bang in the front. Your hair was a constant source of
wonderment to all.

Update: Pocahontas-straight and slightly angled at the face,
or a riot of natural curls.

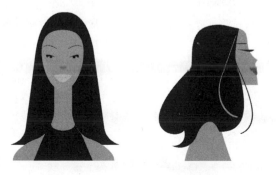

The Ponytail

At its peak: Fifth grade when hair was hot-combed and held at the back with the klik-klak-looking hair holder.

Update: Go for "I Dream of Jeannie" heights with a sexy add-on ponytail.

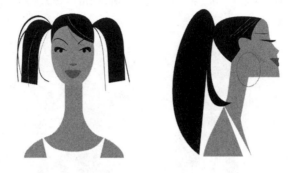

Once you figure out the style that really makes your heart soar, show some photos of the look to your stylist. From there the two of you—before he puts the shears to your mane—should cover the following points:

1. Can your hair—its length, density, and condition—support the look?
2. Is this the most flattering style for your features?
3. Can you afford the maintenance fees—going to the salon every week, chemical touch-up, retwisting, and so on?
4. How much time and effort do you have to invest to keep the hairstyle up?
5. What other options do you have with this particular hairstyle? Can you pull it back in a ponytail? Slick it back? Wave it up?

THINK OUT OF THE BOX

The dollars are short and you need a shot of color or a touch-up. Here are a few suggestions on how to do it yourself and keep your hair. *Warning! Warning!* When using chemicals of any type, really, let a professional do it, but if you're really broke, use the products sparingly and follow the instructions to the letter. What's even better, if you have a friend who is adept at doing hair, enlist her to do yours. And do go overboard with the use of conditioners.

HAIR COLOR

If your hair is already relaxed and you're not going significantly lighter, go with a semi- or demi-permanent color. If you're not experienced with hair color and you want to go significantly lighter than your shade and tone, wait until you get some money and go to your stylist.

If your hair is relaxed, do not use permanent color. I don't care what the box says.

You know the drill: Read the box and the instructions and do the patch test.

If your hair is of medium density, medium curl, shoulder length or shorter, you probably need one box. If your hair is more dense (very thick) or below the shoulder, you need two boxes. It's easier to buy one box more than you think you need. You can always take the box back or save it for touch-ups; better that than to be caught with half your hair done.

On relaxed hair the demi-permanent color will probably last longer (than the usual twenty-four shampoos); because relaxed hair is porous and absorbs more of the color.

Once you color your hair, use a shampoo for color-treated or chemically treated hair, which is gentle and less likely to strip the color.

RELAXERS

When we relax our own hair, one of the biggest mistakes we make is applying the chemicals to the entire hair shaft. If you must straighten at home, keep the following in mind:

1. For touch-ups, always protect your scalp and your skin at the hairline by applying a base of petroleum jelly before you use your relaxer.
2. Saturate previously relaxed hair with a creamy moisturizing conditioner to protect it from the chemicals. And who can't use more conditioning?
3. Always shampoo and rinse one more time to ensure that there is no chemical residue in the hair. Chemical residue can cause irritation and breakage.
4. Work the relaxer through the new growth with your gloved fingers. Do not comb the relaxer through your hair because it will overprocess the previously relaxed hair.
5. Use lye-base relaxers.
6. Never relax and color at the same time, unless bald is the look you're going for.

Yet another thought: I got it, you don't have the money! You may want to inquire at your favorite salon and the more upscale salons about participating in their training nights. A stylist in training is supervised by the licensed professionals in applying relaxers and colors, and in wielding the scissors. Or if you're more adventurous, check out the beauty schools.

MANE TAME

As the world continues to spin on its axis, here are six things that will always be true of our unique strands:

1. There is no such thing as the perfect hairstyle. Black hair is inherently delicate, so it is best to change styles frequently to minimize possible breakage points. For example, whether your hair is natural or relaxed, vary the style—two or three days loose, three or four days twisted or pulled back.

2. Consistent wearing of tight weaves and braids is really a death-to-the-strands sentence. If the braids or the weave offers a secondary benefit like a free face-lift or almond eyes, it is too tight.

3. Tight braids, weaves, and pulled-back hairstyles cause traction baldness.

4. Stretch your relaxer touch-up times from, let's say, six weeks to ten weeks by continually moisturizing and softening new growth with oils, pomades, and/or straightening serums. Always apply serums or anti-frizz pomades on damp hair after shampooing and conditioning so that the drying process will lock in the moisture and the straighter shape of the strand.

5. Wrap hair at night. It will give you a straighter look, cut down on fussing and combing of delicate hair, and protect fragile ends.

6. Invest in a few satin pillowcases or a satin bedcap. Satin doesn't absorb moisture like cotton and its smooth texture will glide over the hair.

Hair Daze

Whether you're swinging from the chandeliers or swinging with another culture abroad, you'll need some guidance on how to keep your hair looking fabulous.

THE MORNING AFTER

It started so innocently. Brotherman asked you out for drinks and conversation and the next thing you know, your best jokes are being told from his bed. That's cool, we're all consenting adults, but damn, aside from the comb in your chic Dior saddle-bag you don't have a thing to take care of your hair. Don't fret. Here are some tips on how to emerge from an all-nighter without your hair looking like the rapper ODB.

Cut is key. Even if you're practicing the Kama Sutra your hair will fall back into place with a little help from a brush or comb. If you're dealing with thug love (a Bro with cornrows), he should have an extra 'do rag. Borrow it and put it on when he puts his on.

Pack a "survival kit." If you go out in the morning not expecting to come back until the dawn, pack a bag. Tote at all times a small plastic baggie with hair elastics or a barrette, a few bobby pins, a trial-size packet of shine serum or oil, moisturizer, holding gel, a silk scarf, and a shower cap swiped from the hotel. Heck, buy multiples of each item and stash them everywhere—in your gym bag and luggage. The hair-care package along with your comb will help you create a quick 'do—a sleek ponytail, bun, or, for shorter hair, seal-slick pixie cut. Natural sisters who are sporting an Afro or a textured 'do should stuff their baggie with a trial-size bottle of leave-in conditioner.

Rummage around Big Poppa's house. Er, well, if you want the relationship to progress, ask first. What can be pressed into a tress saver? Improvise! Check and see if he has a tin of that ever-trusty Murray's Hair Pomade (usually the close-cropped guys own this), or reach for your lip balm (preferably in a tin) like Smith's Rosebud Salve, which can serve as a pomade to sleek hair back and flatten frizzies at the hairline. Shaving cream acts as a mousse and a lifesaver for short- to ear-length re-

laxed hair and natural styles, for it slicks hair down for a Jo
Baker effect. A spritz of Afro Sheen hair sheen if he's not a
baldy. A loud silk tie can be used to wrap around your head as a
stylish alternative to a headband. Or lift one of Brother's
brims—be it a logo'd bucket, Superfly fedora, or a jaunty driv-
ing cap—and rock it!

Global 'Dos

The beautylicious babe is a traveling fool! Work-related jaunts
and exotic vacations send you trotting all over the globe. Don't
let your hair be the passport to a worrisome trip. You have quite
a few style options to consider when going abroad. You can get
your hair braided or opt for flat twists. But what if you don't
want to? What are the options for the relaxed or natural-hair
girl with hair of medium to long length? No matter where you
go, pack the following:

> Blow-dryer with the following: an electrical
>   converter/adaptor that will convert from 110 to 220/240
>   volts; comb or pick attachment; hair bonnet to connect to
>   dryer so that you can set your hair
> Travel-size bottles of holding gel, hair spray, shampoo,
>   moisturizer, a spray bottle of leave-in conditioner, and
>   packets of conditioner
> A baggie of hairpins, bobby pins, barrettes
> A satin cap or pillowcase
> A wig or hairpiece (optional, but great if you know you can't
>   be bothered worrying about your hair at all)

Whether you're in London, Paris, South Africa, or Tokyo, you
still can get your 'do done. You may find yourself on an extended

trip across the Atlantic, or you may be living on a continent other than North America for a while. Don't waste precious time worrying about your hair. Now, of course, don't get carried away. In Africa the stylists don't have a license—which in plain speak means don't let them put any chemicals in your hair! Resist the temptation to buy hair color or relaxer in a foreign country, because the formulations are different. For example, L'Oréal hair color in Japan is different from the Stateside brand in that the formulation is stronger in order for the dye to penetrate Asian hair, which is thicker, more deeply pigmented, and coarser than Caucasian and black hair. Also, you may find products from the United States (the leader in black hair-care products) on the black market, which means that the product's integrity and efficacy are in question—and the relaxer may be as old as you! If you're going to be in a city or country that doesn't have a significant black population, find the U.S. military base and inquire among the Sisters (preferably find the one with a great 'do) about how they maintain their hair. You may luck up on Sistergirl Sergeant who's a stylist, and the on-base convenience store that stocks Ultra Sheen's Gentle Treatment Relaxer and Soft Sheen Optimum Care Relaxer. Of course, if all else fails, you can have your family and friends replenish your supplies monthly. With a few tips and some planning before you go, you can still keep the mane fierce. Below: A look at some of the major international cities and the black hair scene.

LONDON

Yes, the weather is foggy and damp. And the water tends to be hard, particularly if you live in an urban area. What should you have in your Vuitton makeup case? Stow away an antifrizz serum, a cute rain hat, and a clarifying shampoo like Pantene to rid your hair of mineral deposits from the water (which dry and dull the hair).

London is probably second to U.S. cities in terms of know-how, technique, and the overall fabulousness of black hair care. London stylists are known for their outrageous cuts. If you're looking for a good black salon in London, check out the West End and Brixton. Also check out *Black Beauty & Hair* magazine (sold in the States at newsstands that carry foreign mags) or go online to www.blackbeautyandhair.com.

Seek out: The salon and stylist of choice for London's fab girls is Errol Douglas, of the Errol Douglas Salon, located in Belgravia Village, 020 7235 0110.

There are no hard-and-fast rules for tipping. Generally, the shampoo girl gets 1.00 to 2.50 pounds; the senior stylist gets anywhere from 5.00 to 15.00 pounds.

PARIS

In the City of Lights, keep your hair-care regimen simple. Use your basics and a great daily moisturizer to protect your hair from the elements.

If you're looking for the folks, U.S. expatriate and African, hang out in the Passage for flavor and a bevy of black hair salons.

In search of the cutting-edge, fresh-off-the-runway 'do? Well, you need to be in Paris during the shows. The designers show the fall lines at the end of February and spring at the beginning of October.

Once at the show, Ms. Beautylicious should be able to master-key her way backstage, in which case you can ask one of the black hairdressers to do your hair. What's probably easier and more practical for all involved is to hang out where the fashion crowd is (go to the website www.modeaparis.com for fashion schedules) and ask the folks—models, editors, and fashionistas—how you can contact a haute stylist. Most stylists will gladly do your hair and will probably charge you the model rate.

Need a great wash and set? Keep in mind that you're probably not going to get that sassy style that you did at home. Make peace with a good anchorwoman pageboy (for those with shoulder-length or longer, relaxed hair; think a touch fluffier for natural hair), or just plain ole slicked and brushed back, if your hair is ear length or shorter. Truth is, Paris just ain't that fashionable when it comes to black hair. *But,* put function before fashion and you will get a scalp analysis, a clean scalp, and great conditioning treatments, as Paris is the home of some of the best hair-care lines.

Seek out: J. F. Lazartigue, 5 rue faubourg Saint-Honoré, 33 01 42 65 29 24. *Products to covet:* Fab girls Janet Jackson and Tracee Ross are all over the Propolis Gel for itchy scalps and the classic Pre Shampoo Cream, a preconditioning treatment that's loaded with shea butter.

Seek out: Univers-Phyto, located on 104 boulevard Haussmann, 01 45 22 13 14. *Products to covet:* Eve swears by Phytospecific (a plant-based hair-care line made specifically for women of color) like the Vital Force Crème Bath, with nurturing sesame and jojoba oils to baby dry and brittle hair.

Straight talk: Both Lazartigue and Univers-Phyto have hair relaxers, but, again, don't hold them to American standards and expectations. For one thing, they do not use sodium hydroxide. In order to get a touch-up you will need at least four to five inches of new growth. French relaxers will relax the curl some and zap the frizz but won't get hair bone straight. Both shops offer English-speaking stylists of African descent.

SOUTH AFRICA

A burgeoning business spot for savvy African Americans, South Africa is getting rave reviews on its beautiful climate. Again, keeping to your basic hair-care regimen is key. However, you can't go wrong loading up on leave-in conditioners, daily moisturizers, and a couple of great hats. Look to the shopping areas in downtown Capetown and Pretoria for your hair needs. In Capetown, the Clermont and Cavendish Square areas are the places to be. In Pretoria it's Hatfield Square.

Word to the wise: While this is the place to get the most beautifully crafted braids imaginable, think twice. Most of the stylists work out of their home, and due to a bit of unrest, you should consider carefully before venturing out or else find a guide to take you.

Seek out: Don't overlook the hair salon in any of the five-star hotels. Again, keep it simple—wash and set. Do, however, ask the stylist if she does braids in the salon.

TOKYO

Japan is enthralled with all things black. Thus the Japanese youth are thoroughly fascinated with our look. In fact, they have created ways to achieve it for themselves. However, don't go in for the new straightening process that the Japanese have pioneered, because the chemicals will destroy our delicate hair. Really, keep it a wash and set here.

Seek out: The happening area is Shibuya-ku, which is a college town with a SoHo (read real trendy and expensive) vibe. The spots include Aqua.

The truth: As black folks are a seriously tiny minority here, you might want to bring a truckload of your own hair products and start brushing up on your kitchen beautician skills. Or better yet, get your hair braided and enjoy the sights and the people.

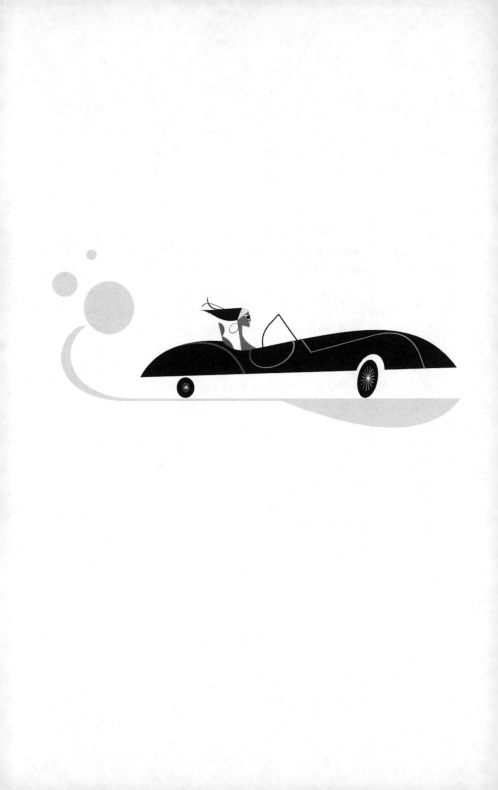

Chapter Seven

Fun and Frolic

*Under pressure people admit to
murder, setting fire to the village church, or
robbing a bank, but never to being a bore.*
—ELSA MAXWELL

*g*o on, cut the fool! Get the bone out of your back. In other words, have fun. The fab girl is not about to spend her time trying to look cool at uptight social events, where everyone looks like they've OD'd on Nytol. Nope, our girl is out telling jokes and is the first one on the dance floor. She knows you don't have to have the wit of Whoopi or Chris Rock to tell a joke, but she's memorized some good ones that she's ready to tell . . . with gusto. The fab girl has no problem hanging out by herself and bringing the noise and the funk with her. The fab girl is a fool for fun and she isn't afraid of looking like one—be it on the golf course or in her attempt to rock the mic. Hey, your new motto: "Whatever it takes to spice things up!"

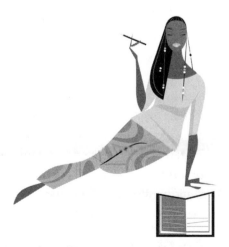

The Bon Vivant

Put your wit and smarts to work in any social situation.

THE TWENTY-FIRST-CENTURY DARK TOWER

> *We dedicate this tower to the aesthetes, that cultured*
> *group of young Negro writers, sculptors, painters,*
> *music artists, composers and their friends.*
> *A place of particular charm.*
> —A'LELIA WALKER

This was the invitation copy for A'Lelia Walker's Dark Tower salon, 1928. Known as the "joy goddess of Harlem's 1920s," A'Lelia Walker (Madam C. J. Walker's daughter) was *the* party giver of the Harlem Renaissance (consider her the precursor to P. Diddy). Her enduring contribution wasn't her lavish, frequently over-the-top shindigs but the literary salon that she hosted for the artists of the day including Langston Hughes, Countee Cullen, Romare Bearden, and Aaron Douglas. She called it the Dark Tower, after Cullen's column in the journal *Opportunity*.

Take a page from A'Lelia's book and run a literary salon out of your home. You don't even have to be an artist. Hey, even A'Lelia said, "Having no talent or gift but a love and keen admiration for art, the Dark Tower was my contribution."

Much more than a book club, the salon fosters camaraderie and can serve as a sounding board for you and your friends' creativity and artistic expression. Make your home the space where folks can get feedback on their poetry, sing in front of an intimate audience, or work out the kinks in their novel among like-minded souls. Not to mention that it's an excellent opportunity for stimulating conversation and meeting new people! Now, your very own Dark Tower needn't be an expensive venture. Consider creating about twenty-five invitations. (Why not send one also to your local "celeb" writers, singers, musicians, and rappers?) Just plump up the cushions on the couch, light some candles, and lay out a spread of crudités, smoked cheese and crackers, buffalo wings (if you're so inclined), and a nice pitcher of homemade iced tea, and let the creativity and conversation flow.

The Jokester

The edict: Make 'em laugh. Your immediate thought? *Eeek!* Now there comes a time when you will be called upon to tell a joke—as an icebreaker at a sales presentation, to keep things light with your boss, to impress the honey at the lounge, or, hell, just because you want to. It really isn't hard. Just keep your good humor and channel your inner Nipsey Russell. Here are some basic tips:

> *Know the joke from start to finish.* If you hear a really good one that you want to tell in the future, jot it down.
> *Focus on the delivery.* The bulk of the joke's success lies in the delivery. Look for something in the joke to embellish, which further engages people and gives them a visual.
> *Finish what you start.* Don't peter out when you encounter a poker face or you feel you've flubbed the punch line.

BOMB SCARE
Nobody laughed? Don't skulk away ashamed and humiliated.

Repeat the punch line loudly. That's not working? Go with Whoopi's technique at the Oscars: Gaze at the befuddled masses and say, "You all will get it next week. It's okay." Of course, you should also laugh real hard and sit down!

Serve Up Hot Chitchat for Dinner

The dinner table conversation is on life support. It's only a matter of seconds before someone deals the death blow by asking in a bored monotone, "Uhmm . . . Did you say that your name is Ashanti? What does that mean in Swahili?" or the cringe-worthy favorite, "Uhmm . . . Do you think it's going to rain?" Be prepared to resuscitate the conversation and add a few sparks with some off-the-wall questions: "If they sent you to Pluto, what five CDs would you take with you and why?" "Is Jay-Z the musical genius of our time?" (This really ought to get the conversation heated!) Or go for the shoe personality test: Come up with analyses of folks' kicks. I don't need to tell you to keep it sweet. For example, *stilettos* mean the wearer is a sexy gal trying to add a little height to her life. But don't go here: a man's gray loafers mean he's a broken-down wanna-be player. Remember, the goal of dinner conversation is to keep things moving and fun. Hostility is not an option. If the conversation has flat-lined, you can always excuse yourself and go to the powder room!

Going Soul-O

Sometimes the best adventures are those in which you go prowling the streets by yourself, sans your girls. Just follow your gut and pinpoint a spot. It may be someplace you've always wanted

to go—that is, a new restaurant, gallery, museum, or seminar—
or you may have the bug to walk aimlessly around town. At any
rate, all you need to take to have a good time is an open mind and
childlike curiosity. And remember, smile and chat up the natives.
You can always use another friend!

At a loss for new barriers to break by your lonesome?
Nonsense! The beautylicious babe is full of ideas on finding fun,
herself, and possibly a new beau, alone. Why don't you:

1. *Walk on the wild side.* Live in the suburbs or the yuppified
   section of the city? Take a stroll through the ghettos
   (shame on you if you automatically thought *black*!). Nope,
   the ghetto is defined by Webster's as a quarter of a city in
   which members of a minority group live. So stroll
   through Chinatown, Little Italy, and Little Russia. Try
   the food; walk around and observe the people and their
   customs. And, for all of you who think Harlem, Compton,
   and Newark are to be driven through with the windows
   up and the doors locked, it's time to get out of your car
   and take a stroll to reacquaint yourself with the folks, the
   food, and the flavor of the 'hood.

2. *Discover new shopping haunts.* Scout the cute out-of-the-
   way vintage stores for the original inspiration of a piece
   you're pining for. For example, if you're craving a sexy,
   bold print top, why not troll the vintage shops and flea
   markets for Pucci or Leonard's of Paris designs? An
   evening bag? Look for ladylike sequined framed bags. Or
   slide through the ethnic shops that sell traditional
   African, Indian, or Asian clothes, accessories, jewelry, and
   art, and get inspired.

3. *Taste different varieties of the grape.* Many liquor stores
   have free wine-tasting classes. Why not finally learn the

difference between a burgundy and a pinot noir? Find out about tastings by inquiring at your local liquor store. Uhm, a tip: Don't embarrass yourself by asking at the spot that Ned the wino frequents; look to the liquor stores in the more upscale part of town. Also check out the website www.wines-across-america.com for vineyards near you, or check out the wine lovers' page at www.wine-lovers-page.com.

4. *Check out the opera.* Start with either a classic story like Bizet's *Carmen* or Puccini's *Madame Butterfly,* where you have a bit of an idea about the plotline. You know you're a sucker for passion, love, and murder, all done loudly! Or check out the opera that stars fellow fabulites like mezzo-soprano Denyse Graves and those legends Jessye Norman and Kathleen Battle.

5. *Saunter into a jazz club.* Don a sexy outfit and sidle up to the bar for a cocktail and some cool jazz. Let your curiosity and your taste guide you as to whether you want to hear jazz vocalists, Afro-Latin, swing, or bebop. The subgenres of jazz are too overwhelming? Hey, there's no shame in your game if you let the lure of the delectable jazz musician help you make a choice. You can't go wrong with any Marsalis, Roy Hargrove, or Joshua Redman.

6. *See divas live!* Go see the legendary Dolls perform when they come to town. Immerse yourself in old-school glamour and watch the Dolls trill and thrill. Let's face it, though, this isn't going to be everyone's cup of tea. You say *icon,* your friends say *fossil.* Well, what do they know? Grab a front-row seat for Diahann Carroll doing the theater, Eartha Kitt kicking up at the Carlyle, Darlene Love and Freda Payne on the cabaret circuit, or Donna Summer and Diana Ross on the concert circuit. Surround yourself with true aficionados and have a blast!

7. *Rent a convertible.* To hell with your
   hair! Rent or borrow a convertible and
   hit the open road. Feel the wind through
   your mane, the sun on your shoulders,
   and just drive. Pure exhilaration!

8. *Take a seminar or a college course.* Learn something new.
   Take art history or a literature class to find out what Toni
   Morrison really meant in *Beloved.* Or you can make it fun,
   practical, and wacky. Why not take an auto mechanic
   course or singing lessons to satisfy your inner mezzo-
   soprano?

9. *Lie around in the lap of luxury.* This one is fun when
   you're feeling particularly flush and you can't stand
   another moment of your messy flat. Go to a neighboring
   city and stay a night at the poshest hotel. Call room
   service, or better yet, get dressed and have din-din or
   cocktails at the hotel's restaurant or bar.

10. *Loll around at a destination spa.* Take a weekend to get
    back in the groove of eating right and exercising along
    with some serious pampering.

Now, Voyager

> *Darling!!! What you need in life is a passport.*
> —AUDREY SMALTZ

Take the fabulous legendary fashion authority Audrey Smaltz's
advice and get yourself a passport. And if you have one, use it
more regularly! Why? Travel is one of the best ways to broaden
your education and your perspective on the world. It increases
your understanding of other peoples and cultures. You will experience firsthand breathtaking views and historic landmarks

and you'll learn how to adapt to new climes and people. The side benefit is that travel makes you a more interesting person and it also amps up your confidence, especially if you travel alone. Take a plane beyond your usual getaways to Jamaica or the Bahamas and start hopping about to far-flung places. Hell, start visiting other states. So go, mingle, eat the local food, learn the language, and take in the beauty of the country's architecture and the countryside. Six ideas to get your motor running:

1. *Drive cross-country with your girls.* Grab a map and go from east to west or north to south. Best to do right after college when you have the time and the tolerance.

2. *Try an unusual island.* There are other islands in the Caribbean beyond Barbados, the Bahamas, and Bermuda. Check out Bonaire, a beautiful, quiet (that is, it's not a tourist trap) Dutch Caribbean island known for its snorkeling and scuba diving.

3. *Jet to Paris for the weekend.* Monitor the travel section for great fares to Paris. Use the Twinkie Theorum (page 22) and close your eyes and charge it.

4. *Designate your birthday for special destinations.* Quick! Throw out five places you've always wanted to go and write them down. Don't censor the list because you feel it's outlandish or it's impossible. Safari in Kenya? Hey, make that next year's birthday gift. Let your friends in on the fun and see who wants to go. Now begin your Send Me Away savings account at the bank. Make weekly deposits. Get geeked up by gathering information on a trip to Kenya and scanning prices weekly. Make reservations for a trip next year.

5. *Party on.* Experience new ways to shake it up and shake your tail feathers. That may be Carnaval in Brazil or

Europe's biggest street fest, Notting Hill Carnival in
London.

6. *Join a travel group.* Check out your alumni association,
church, or social club so that you can travel to exotic
locales with like-minded people. The good thing about a
travel group is that generally you have a knowledgeable
guide who can point out the landmarks and areas of
interest.

Dream and doodle with these sites and magazines:

www.concierge.com
www.travelnotes.org
www.cheapvacationsonline.com
www.expedia.com
Holiday Magazine and *Travel & Leisure* magazine

Cinema Beautylicious

Movies are the stuff that fuels dreams, transports minds and
hearts, and, of course, makes one laugh, cry, or just yawn. But
for the beautylicious babe, movies are the stuff of glorious inspiration. And a good reason to break out a bottle of champagne
and a box of chocolate truffles! Here, a list of the beautylicious
babe's Twenty Must-Own Movies:

1. *Mahogany:* Other than the fact that this flick stars the
incomparable patron saint of fabulosity, Diana Ross, fab
girls young and old will totally relate to our tenacious
heroine's climb from ghetto to continental glamour. But
the clincher really is that girlfriend held tight to her

dreams of being a designer, even if it did mean leaving a very fine Billy Dee Williams, who was an activist lawyer to boot. Fashion, doe eyes, and the line "Success is nothing without someone you love to share it with" make this the fab girl's number one pick.

2. *Carmen Jones:* The beauteous Dorothy Dandridge turns this mutha out. Get out your pads and take notes 'cause no one could work a room like Miss Carmen. Lusty, sultry, and passionate, she drives her men to distraction (always a nice skill to have) and, well, murder. A fab girl favorite because of Carmen's steaminess and the blinding beauty of DD and her costar, Harry Belafonte. Passion should always look this good.

3. *Breakfast at Tiffany's:* While the gamine appeal of Audrey Hepburn wasn't a big issue to us, we loved the insouciance, the clothes, and, yes, the Holly Golightly-ness of it all. The beautylicious babe is all about Holly's "itness."

4. *Sparkle:* The Supreme-like group (Irene Cara, Lonette McKee, and Dwan Smith) represent the different facets of the beautylicious girl. Lonette McKee is wild, impetuous, and beautiful. Dwan Smith came on as a quiet fire, smart and deeply sensitive. And little Irene Cara shone as loyal, generous, loving, and willfully naïve. Sequins, big hair, dangerously sexy men, and the Curtis Mayfield sound track make this a classic.

5. *Imitation of Life:* C'mon, Sara Jane (Pecola, played by beautylicious icon Fredi Washington in the original 1934 version) was a pistol. So light that she can pass for white, Sara Jane treats her sainted dark-skinned mother like, er, the maid, simply because she thinks that white skin is synonymous with a good life and, damn it, she wants a good life with a good blond husband. It is somewhat archaic now—and I say *somewhat* because we all know that there is

some very unfab black girl who still buys into this notion—
but the fab girl loves the tearjerker aspect of this story
immensely. The loving, self-sacrificing ma whose only crime
is that she couldn't bestow white status or for that matter
manners on her daughter, and the rude, misguided Sara
Jane make for a fascinating dynamic. The scene of scenes, of
course, is Ma's grand New Orleans–style funeral procession
in which Sara Jane runs tearfully behind the horse-drawn
carriage crying, "Mama, Mama." It still gets the tears
flowing.

6. *Coffy; Foxy Brown:* Beautylicious icon Pam Grier's
   message is simple: Ya gotta know when and how to kick
   butt. Fab girls drink in Coffy because of her sensational
   Afro, bod, and attitude. Anyway, like the beautylicious
   babe, Foxy's "A whole lotta woman!"
   Honorable mention—*Cleopatra Jones:* Tamara Dobson as
   Cleo brought elegance to this raunchy genre, but where is
   she now?

7. *Eve's Bayou:* Beautylicious dolls Lynn Whitfield and
   Debbi Morgan strut their stuff in this classy drama
   directed by Kasi Lemmons. Visually stunning, our girls
   mesmerize in their divine fifties frocks and fierce
   demeanors: Lynn is at her elegant, high-strung best,
   while perennially cute Debbi works her mysterious,
   warm, and witchy wiles. And don't forget Diahann going
   very unglam as the voodoo woman.

8. *She's Gotta Have It:* Whatever Nola wants, Nola gets.
   Our precursor to *Sex in the City,* this Spike Lee–directed
   vehicle was one of the first films to show the
   beautylicious babe going for hers sexually without shame.
   Girlfriend is running with three dramatically different
   suitors and is in no real rush to give any of them up. We
   say bravo!

9. *Othello:* Iago and the gang may hate the Moor, but the fab girl loves her Shakespeare, especially when the delectable Laurence Fishburne is reciting the Bard.

10. *Love and Basketball: Ahh,* our kind of love story. Lovely Sanaa Lathan is a female basketball player who plays hard and fast for her man's heart without compromising what she is. With a cast that includes fab girl faves like chocolate goody Omar Epps, cutie pie Debbi Morgan, graceful Alfre Woodard, and fab girl director Gina Prince-Bythewood at the helm, the movie celebrates the sneaky slam dunk of love.

11. *Boomerang:* Director Reggie Hudlin put together a pantheon of fabulosity: the patron saint Eartha Kitt, madcap Grace Jones, icy glam Robin Givens, and the ever-luminous Halle Berry all get together in this saucy comedic romp.

12. *What's Love Got to Do With It:* In this film, based on the real-life story of fab icon Tina Turner, the ever-fabulous Angela Bassett turns in the performance of a lifetime as the abused soul survivor. A little-known fact is that the wigs are the costars. Check it out; when Sir Laurence's Ike dons the Beatles' mop top and Anna Mae is hiding out in Cher-length falls, you don't need any dialogue to know that these two have hit rock bottom (literally).

13. *Clueless:* This frothy little comedy about a blond Beverly Hills princess could well have been a turnoff, but Alicia Silverstone's Cher is just adorable. The clothes, the lingo, and the willful airheadedness are all good-natured fun. Best of all, real-life Ms. Beautylicious Stacey Dash plays Cher's equally vapid sidekick, Dionne, with aplomb. A total Betty, girlfriend gets extra points for playing sweet sixteen and looking it, although in actuality she was far

from it. Honorable mention: *Legally Blonde*. The beautylicious babe understands being underestimated. Plus, Reese Witherspoon is way cool.

14. *Love Jones:* Brother lays eyes on you and now he's reciting poetry about the image of you. Hello! Sign us up. Pretty little Nia Long plays a sexy photographer and "whoa he's cute" Larenz Tate is Mr. Poetryman, with a smile and a way with words guaranteed to melt any woman's heart. The depiction of the hits and misses of this young black love hookup is one of the best to hit the silver screen. Honorable mention: *Jason's Lyric:* It's all about Jada Pinkett Smith and Allen Payne's sensual encounter.

15. *Coming to America:* Yep, this was every beautylicious babe's dream at one point. To have some wonderful, humble, attractive Brother approach you with respect, shower you with kindness and understanding, and then reveal he's really a prince (or at least an NBA draft pick), and, after a bit of tension, you get to have the lavish wedding you've wanted since age five. Kudos to actress Shari Headley (where is she? she was positively gorgeous!) and Eddie Murphy for getting into our heads and getting it right.

16. *All About Eve:* The lesson of this classic 1950 movie? Watch your back, there is always somebody ready to step into your shoes. Bette Davis plays actress Margo Channing, who has everything and now nothin' because her understudy, Eve (Anne Baxter), is appropriating her life, right down to moving in on her man. Fasten your seatbelt, because this movie is going to be a bumpy and wonderfully bitchy ride.

17. *The Women:* The beautylicious babe enjoys a bitch fest, especially when it's laced with sharp dialogue from

renaissance woman and wit Clare Boothe Luce. Although the 1939 flick centers on "friends" gossiping about a straying husband and his perfect wife, you never see any men. Look for Joan Crawford as the conniving counter girl.

18. *What Ever Happened to Baby Jane?:* Joan Crawford and Bette Davis are going at it in this over-the-top drama about two dysfunctional sisters. Joan's crippled because of Bette's arrested development and hatred. Whoa . . . these broads go at it better than Tyson and Holyfield.

19. *Claudine:* The ever-elegant Diahann Carroll goes ghetto as a welfare mother who falls in love with the garbage man played by James Earl Jones. The role garnered Diahann an Oscar nomination for best actress in 1974.

20. *Monster's Ball:* You have to ask? Halle turned it out and won the Academy Award for Best Actress, an award that had eluded us for seventy-four years.

Game Tight

Break into a few of the boy bastions of fun. Here are some tips so that you can go from clueless rookie to MVP.

BILLIARDS AND THE BEAUTYLICIOUS BABE

True, pool has always seemed to be a game suited for the femme fatale. You can lean over the cue stick seductively to show mean cleavage. You can prop your hips seductively on the pool table to position yourself for a particular ball. There is no end to the posing that can go on with pool, but the biggest turn-on may be that you can actually play. Get into the proper form: balanced stance, legs comfortably apart, head bent over the cue stick. Your grip should be firm but not tight, with the thumb, index, and middle finger, and on the handle of the cue stick, not on the "butt plate," which is the end of the stick. Your arm is perpendicular to the floor. The other hand forms a bridge to guide the cue stick—that is, the heel of the hand and last three fingers are on the table, thumb and index finger circling the stick. The end of the stick should be eight inches from the white cue ball.

Firmly spank that ball. Where you contact the ball affects how it spins and where on the table it stops spinning. For solid contact the center is the ideal place to hit. Above center, and the cue ball will spin forward or keep rolling after it hits the contact ball (you know, the striped or solid-colored ball). Below center, it'll "draw" and stop dead on contact. "English" means hitting the left or right side of the cue ball for sidespin. "Bank" shots are when you ricochet the cue ball off the cushion to make your shot. When do you need the chalk? Well, think of the cue as an emery board; after an hour of use it gets smooth and loses its grab. Chalk gives the friction you need to hit without slipping. That way you won't "scratch" or screw up the shot by slipping off the cue ball so that it rolls about an inch.

ALWAYS BET ON BLACK . . . JACK!

Whether you're in Atlantic City, Vegas, or Monte Carlo, nothing says gambling with a capital G quite like the blackjack table. Forgo the zombie position at the slot machine and really get into the spirit of the game by playing blackjack. First off, know that even though there are other players at the table, you're only betting against the dealer to see whose cards add up to twenty-one or closest to it without going over and losing. Face cards count as ten. An ace is either a one or an eleven—it's your call. To "hit" (take another card), tap or scratch the felt behind the cards. To "stand" (no more cards), wave your hand once over the cards. A few tips for playing like a pro:

> If the dealer is showing a six or less and you have thirteen or more, stand. The dealer must hit on anything up to sixteen and the odds are he will go over twenty-one.
>
> Knowing which pairs to split is a complicated decision, but if you don't split eights or aces people will look at you funny (sixteen is a piss-poor hand; eight is more promising). Separate the cards side by side and place another equal-sized bet beside your first one. Then indicate to the dealer to either stand or (unless you've split aces) hit again.
>
> Always double your bet when you have an eleven. Put the chip beside the original bet.

TEE TIME

You've heard that the golf course is where the monied honeys are and now you're ready to go clubbin'. Not so fast, Ms. Frisky, let's hit the greens with a clue. Golf is more than a chance to prance around in a color-coordinated visor, Izod polo, Lily Pulitzer shorts, and your lovely bronzed legs. Toots, you won't even be a distraction. Golf is a game of intense concentration and spare, controlled motions. You can still be a fun fourth by keeping these points in mind: (1) Don't slow the game down and (2) Don't mess up the other players. (That is, kill the loud talking, laughing, and O. J. Simpson–type narration.) At tee-off time, don't tee off the other players. Talking when someone's about to swing at the ball is a major no-no, and never stand behind another player. If your ball curves left, you've hit a "hook." If it veers right it's a "slice" or "banana." A ball that barely gets off the tee is a "worm burner." Take a "mulligan"; that's a do-over. On the fairway, always replace your divots: Put back any chunks of sod you hack up. When you close in on the green you'll need your pitching wedge to hit out of the tall grass and then your putter to go for the hole. When you go to putt, leave the wedge on the "pin" that's been pulled out of the cup and left on the apron (the grass around the green). On the the green, don't drop your bag or cross the "lines" between the player's ball and the cup. If your ball is in the way of someone else's, "mare" it by replacing it with a coin until it's your turn.

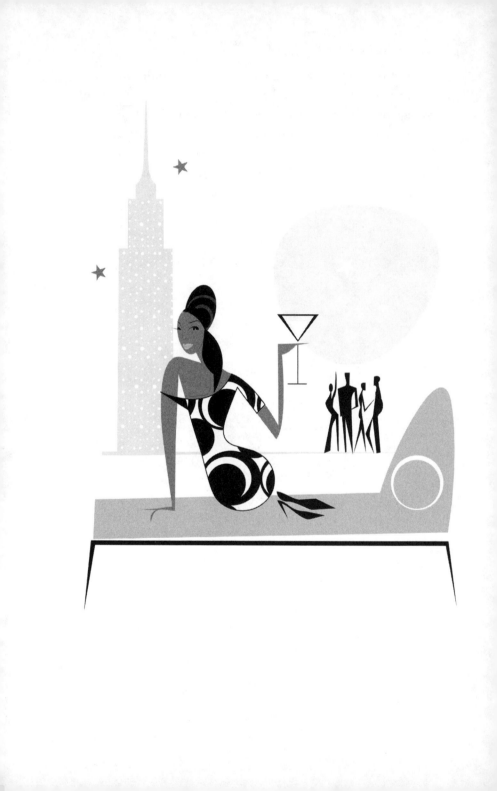

Chapter Eight

Fête Accompli

I made people feel welcome and at home.
They enjoyed my entertaining, but that wasn't
the main reason why they came.
They liked the atmosphere I created.
—BRICKTOP

hrow the doors open to your domicile. The word is out: For fun, laughs, and good times you're a pretty hard act to beat. Parlay your rep as a good-time girl (and I mean that in the most flattering sense of the word) into hostess extraordinaire. Entertaining and/or throwing a party need not be a stiff, anal affair. I am not talking about those "bourgie" affairs, where the hostess is so focused on her nouvelle soul cuisine and the appropriate showcasing of her Waterford crystal and Lenox china that she fails to notice that everyone is politely bored. No, you can move the crowd with the five Cs: cuisine, cocktails, confidence, cheerfulness, and a dash of comedy.

Dinner Dynamics

THE KITCHEN MAGICIAN (OR HOW TO MAKE TAKEOUT WORK FOR YOU)

The new Loveman is coming over for dinner at 8 P.M. tonight. You're still sitting at work at 6 P.M. with nothing but a flat Diet Coke and a can of tuna. Don't cry. Pick up the phone and order takeout from your favorite soul food restaurant. Or run past the home-style fast-food joints like Boston Market. Consider the supermarket for a rotisserie chicken and a few shotgun sides like mashed potatoes or macaroni salad. Once home, season the store-bought macaroni salad with season salt and maybe some crunchy vegetable, 'cause we all know that the store salads are as bland as they come and that would blow your cover.

FABULOUS DINING

Five ways to take an ordinary dining experience and make it an event:

+ Using the good china and the lovely linen napkins from Grandma for your franks and beans
+ Gathering the remains of the roses at your local florist at the end of the day and scattering them on the table, on the floor, or on your bed before he comes over
+ Replacing your regular kitchen lightbulb with a sexy soft pink light, for ambiance
+ Using warm washcloths and slices of lemon to clean off your hands after your meal
+ Splurging on the most decadent chocolate cake you can find

Party People Incorporated

The gang is gathering at your place tonight at eight? No problem. Check out a few thematic solutions to "Looks like a Blockbuster night."

THE GAMING ROOM

Throw a pot of turkey chili on the stove and artfully arrange the nachos and the salsa on the table. Break out a deck of cards and take it back to the dorm days with a roaring good game of cards like Bid Whist or Spades and plenty of gossip. Or turn the old school games from your attic into some new fun. Is it a boys and girls gathering? Get twisted out on Twister. Let the wine and beer flow and go for what you know on the blue circle! Don't sleep on the "What am I going to be?" games like Life and Monopoly. Break them out and start talking much smack about what you're going to do with Park Place or when the spin of the Life wheel tells you to skip college and get married. Another game that requires a lot of imagination and a lot of liquor is Mystery Date. If you can find this moldy oldie cop it quick! The basic premise of this board game is to get

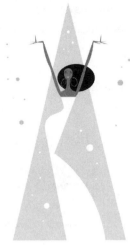

your dream man—the jock, the prom king—and avoid the nerd. Yes, the guys are, ahem, white. And no, no one looks like Brad Pitt, but the beauty of this game is mentally replacing the white archetypes with some Brothers that everyone can agree on (can we say Morris Chestnut?), be they guys from Lit 101 or famous. That's when the fun begins!

THE JURASSIC PARK JAM

Remember when all things good were def and Eric B nominated his deejay for president? Still pining for one nation under a groove? If so, it's time to throw the old school party. No you don't need Funkmaster Flex to make this happen. Make a couple of mix tapes. The cheapest way is to tape straight off your local hip-hop or R&B station, usually around noon or Friday night when they typically go for a trip down memory lane. Or, for a couple of dollars, slip a few tapes or blank CDs to the neighborhood deejay so that he can dig in the crates for everyone from the Cold Crush Crew to Chuck Brown and the Soul Searchers to the Notorious BIG. Take 'em back to yesteryear with the jeans, sneakers, and gold-chain dress code. Send invites in the shape of a Kangol hat or Adidas sneaker. The drink of choice, Olde E from the bodega and bottles of hard lemonade. Snack on with barbecue and onion-garlic potato chips and fried chicken wings. Be warned: this is a party that's gonna make you sweat!

In the Spirits

Urban Negroes are becoming more "urbane." Every day more emphasis is being placed on "gracious living." Consumption patterns are advancing toward a greater acceptance of the cocktail preferences of the sophisticate. Brandy and Cognac producers can effectively take advantage of this trend toward more elegant, yet leisurely, living by advertising these liqueurs of the smart set—whom the masses emulate.

—*EBONY* AND *JET* MAGAZINE, 1957

That's you, doll, sexy, urbane, and a devout practitioner of the art of gracious living. Make it your civic duty to bring back the cocktail hour. Let 'em know that mirth and cheer live here with the clinking of martini glasses, for you are the sensuous alchemist, that sexy creature who's able to blend fiery spirits into intoxicating potions that soothe the mind, body, and soul. Create a mood, cast a spell, and stir up a conversation with a cosmopolitan. It's everything from Manolos and martinis to love and scotch on the rocks. Take a tip from fab icon Lena Horne, who presided gleefully over her experimental cocktail hour on Saturdays and Sundays. She would read her trusty cocktail book and try a different recipe from the book every weekend until she had prepared every drink listed at least once. Stand back and marvel at how your place has now become a haven for all things good: friends, drinks, conversation, and music. While immersed in all things boozy, learn your limits. Walk on the sane side of tipsy, so that you can keep the party rocking and the threat of blackmail nonexistent. This is your moment, Babe, pour some Henny on it! Here's how:

BAR FLY

A well-stocked bar is your secret weapon. You don't have to spend your whole paycheck on liquor (especially after you gave Jimmy Choo most of your dough), but you can buy a few of the essentials first and swing back for the specialty ingredients.

Essentials

HAVE AT LEAST ONE BOTTLE
OF EACH ON HAND:
Champagne
White wine
Red wine
Vodka
Rum
Gin

Champagne and wine are the elixirs of the romantic evening, the celebratory event, and just plain ole home alone. For more on champagne see the Luxe Life chapter (page 181). Vodka, rum, and gin are classic mixers that can go with the beverages you already have in the fridge, that is, Diet Coke, Pepsi, orange juice, and water. These are simple get-blitzed-quick drinks that are guy-friendly and are also friendly to your girl who's spilling her guts with her latest he-done-me-wrong song.

Gearing up to throw a party? Stock up on the essentials and throw these into the mix:

Tequila
Brandy
Your favorite liqueur, i.e., toasted almond, coffee, or chocolate

Tequila, with the help of crushed ice and lime juice, is the oomph in a margarita, and thus is a real party starter. Brandy connotes a quiet, sophisticated evening. A warm, full-bodied drink, brandy stands best alone.

COOL TOOLS

Since there will be a whole lot of shaking going on, you will need the following gizmos and widgets:

Ice bucket: Nothing says get your drink on quite like this glamorous party accessory. Make sure you have one, be it a psychedelic plastic unit or a chichi glass bucket.

Cocktail shaker: Shades of Sammy Davis Jr., the martinis will be flowing with this classic contraption. The standard shaker comes with a tumbler, built-in strainer, and fitted cap.

Bar spoon: A long skinny spoon with a twisted handle that is used for stirring tall noncarbonated drinks.

Citrus juicer: Stop leaning on Dole and Tropicana. Making drinks with fresh juice separates the pros from the wanna-bes. Your glass reamer is great for the occasional drink, but if you're aiming for hostess with the mostest, invest in an electric juicer. Tip: Increase the amount of juice you get from the fruit by rolling it on a flat surface or warming it with hot water.

Glasses

Have at least four of the following drinking glasses on hand:

Champagne: Narrow flute-shaped stemmed glasses keep the
champagne bubbly longer.

Wineglasses: Stemmed glasses with plenty of room allow the
wine to breathe.

Brandy: Wide bottom and narrow top allow the brandy to be
swirled around to oxygenate it.

Martini: Wide-rimmed, long-stemmed, V-shaped glasses are
the traditional shape.

Liquor: Tumblers with plenty of room to add mixers and ice.

Shot: Essential for measuring your booze.

What's beyond fabulous? If you're having a really big
shindig, say a formal dinner or a big party, hire the cute bartender from the neighborhood watering hole to keep the joy
juice jumping. Sounds like a needless expense, but factor in that
you'll have your mind reeling with dinner, witty banter, and
who needs to be separated from whom, and it's a few dollars
well spent. Look to paying the cute bartender about twenty dollars an hour (in most big cities).

LUSH-IOUS YOU

The empress of elixirs (that's you, sweetie!) emerges from her
boudoir ready to create magic. When dressing for her cocktail
parties she has only three rules: The lips are lacquered, the drag
is sexy but comfy, and the personality is as fizzy as a just-opened
bottle of Moët & Chandon. She may don an ensemble like Lena
Horne's, a fitted but comfortable silk blouse (think vintage
Pucci), unbuttoned to show a bit of cleavage. Fitted slim slacks
and mules (change into ballet slippers when the feet start

squealing), or languorous silk pajamas for the informal do. The soiree of soirees (yours or someone else's), of course, calls for serious dress-up. Summon up your inner Holly Golightly and work a slinky little black dress, paired with killa heels, and accessorize with some sparklies and a smile.

IMBIBE, SHE SAID

There's a drink for every time and place. The fab girl lives for the fun and challenge of matching the appropriate libations to the occasion. The keys are creating mood and experimenting. The coolest kitty will develop her own signature drink. And, hey, don't be afraid to take your mix-master skills out on the road. Instead of the old "I'll bring the chips" attitude, surprise your friends with the ingredients to mix up a batch of your special brew.

It's you and the crew on Saturday afternoon. You're about to pop *Mahogany* in the VCR and let loose some good gossip. Pep up the hen fest with pallie Charlotte's version of the margarita, which is guaranteed to loosen lips. Works better than truth serum.

Charlotte's Gabarita

3 OUNCES GOOD-QUALITY GOLD TEQUILA

1½ OUNCES FRESHLY SQUEEZED LIME JUICE

1½ OUNCES FRESHLY SQUEEZED LEMON JUICE

2 TEASPOONS CONFECTIONERS' SUGAR

Mix ingredients in cocktail shaker. Pour into martini glasses and garnish with strawberries or raspberries.

Serves four

Nibbles

Fast-food heaven—pizza, or a sack full of White Castle burgers and fries.

Beautylicious Mimosa

Great anytime and so very easy: Purée four cups of fresh strawberries in the blender. Fill four champagne flutes with a 1/3 cup of champagne and then pour in strawberry purée. Garnish with a slice of strawberry.

Nibbles

Darling, we demand the best! Jumbo shrimp with cocktail sauce, mini quiche bits, and skewered grilled chicken with a teriyaki sauce.

IF THERE'S A CURE FOR THIS . . .

You want it! The Boss may be crooning on about her love hangover, but trust, there ain't nothing sweet or cute about an alky hangover. Jackhammer pounding headaches and visions of pink elephants dancing through your head aren't the way to start the new morn. The best way to avoid the moanin' after is with a few preventive strikes:

- ✦ Abstain from the grain. Yeah, now let's get real.
- ✦ Eat before swilling. Downing a handful of onion and garlic potato chips beforehand doesn't count. Chow down on high-fiber foods or fatty foods, which break down the alcohol and absorb it.
- ✦ Pop a vitamin C tablet. Studies find that this cold fighter also may guard against hangovers.
- ✦ Drink plenty of water before going to bed.

If the damage has already been done, take the bite out of your bender by drinking lots of water—which cleanses and hydrates—followed with a nonsteroidal, anti-inflammatory painkiller like Tylenol.

BEAUTYLICIOUS BELIEF: Girls, take my word for it: If your job involves socializing, you need to know a few cute drinks to order when you're out with the boss and clients. Learn from my shame. I was about to seal the deal with the client—a VP at a renowned hair-care company. My boss is the president of a high-flying beauty public relations outfit. And we were at one of the playgrounds of the rich and powerful, the Four Seasons bar in New York City. Everything was going great until the bartender asked what everyone would be drinking. The boss went trendy with a dirty martini, the client went urbane alpha male with scotch and water, and your friend just went high school with a Singapore Sling. Hell, I couldn't think of anything else; I'm not a big drinker. Bottled water sounded like a stale teetotaler, vodka and cranberry juice sounded like a rough broad. Champagne, a bit pretentious. Yikes!! Oh, the mirth and jokes that order provided! I wanted to dissolve into the drink, but I learned a lesson. Image counts. Clear down to liquor. Don't get caught looking like a liquor novice. Always have a hot drink (like the Cuban mojito) and a classic (the always-right martini) in your repertoire of drinks. Neither the boss nor the client needs to know of your preference for Alizé, Olde E, or rotgut. You can keep up with the trendy drinks by hitting the hippest lounge or bar in your town for a monthly taste testing and/or befriending the previously mentioned cute bartender.

Libation Songs

Create that mellow, kind of groovy vibe that makes the cocktails go down easier. Here are twenty albums that swing:

1. *Gershwin for Lovers* (Columbia), Marcus Roberts
2. *Belly of the Sun* (Blue Note), Cassandra Wilson
3. *The Girl from Ipanema, The Antonio Carlos Jobim Songbook* (Polygram), various artists
4. *Eartha Kitt Live at the Plaza* (7N), Eartha Kitt
5. *Jazzmatazz Vol. 1* (Capital), Guru
6. *Lady in Satin* (Sony), Billie Holiday
7. *The Essential Dinah Washington,* The Great Songs (Polygram)
8. *Afro-Roots* (Prestige), Mongo Santamaria
9. *The Wham of Sam* (Warner Archives), Sammy Davis Jr.
10. *Volume 17, Verve Jazz Masters* (Polygram), Nina Simone
11. *Mama's Gun* (Universal) Erykah Badu
12. *One Step Forward* (Higher Octave), Les Nubians
13. *Sarah Vaughan with Clifford Brown* (Polygram)
14. *Big Calm* (Sire), Morcheeba
15. *Best of Sade* (Sony)
16. *Verve Remixed* (Universal), various artists
17. *To the Ends of the Earth* (Fantasy), Freddy Cole
18. *John Coltrane and Johnny Hartman* (Grp Records)
19. *Pass the Peas: The Best of the J.B.'s* (Polygram)
20. *A Swingin' Affair!* (Capitol), Frank Sinatra

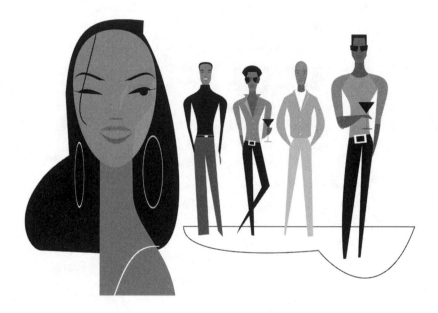

Chapter Nine

Date-o-Rama

*No time to marry, no time to settle
down; I'm a young woman and
ain't done runnin' round.*
—BESSIE SMITH

*H*oney Bunny, you're much too fly to be sitting in the house on Saturday night. The beautylicious babe isn't going to let the urban myth about the Brother shortage—they're either imprisoned, married, or gay—stop her from getting her groove on. She knows how to increase her odds. This determined huntress takes action. She doesn't wait for Mr. Right to knock at her apartment door, 'cause she knows that will be one mighty long and lonely wait. Nope, she gets out and kicks it up 'cause she's in love with life. Yes, you're cute, smart, and funny, but are you game tight? Sorry to sound like a bore, but get out there and hang out, experiment, and play with a lot of different guys. Let the steamy Carmen Jones and others teach you how to sharpen your womanly wiles. Learn how to move out of your comfort zone and also when to call it quits. And, girl, while you're at it, sharpen your gaydar so that you're clear on who's good for hitting the sheets and who's good for sitting through *La Traviata*. In the words of the immortal William "Smokey" Robinson's mama, "You better shop around." Dating helps you figure out what you want and don't want in a partner. Get out of thinking

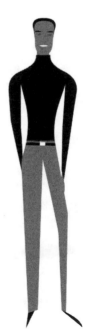

that every potential beau needs to be marriage material. Give yourself options and have a ball (literally and figuratively)!

Flirt Alert

After all, flirting is nothing more than a celebration of your fabulous self.

FAB ARTILLERY

What's the secret to grabbing Brother's attention and keeping it? A hint: It's not your La Perla underpinnings, the tight Earl jeans that encase your world-class booty, or strands you feel are worthy of a shampoo commercial. While those things can help, it really boils down to three behaviors that can't be bought:

1. *Laughter:* What can be cooler than a doll who shows that she can be amused? Laughing is the fab way of always saying that you are delighted with the man's company. Laughter is a joyful, magnanimous response that puts everyone at ease. Unless of course, you're laughing at someone, which is a very unfab, *très* gauche thing to do. The beautylicious babe giggles, chuckles, and, hell, if the joke is a killer diller, guffaws. In other words, she lets him know she's enjoying the moment and his presence.
2. *Looking:* The beautylicious babe makes eye contact. She gives him full attention when he's talking. And whether he's a love man or the handyman, she never looks past him to see if something better is strutting by.
3. *Listening:* The beautylicious babe is all about being a captive audience, because Brotherman is truly interesting, or she's got to pay attention to ascertain that he actually

isn't. At any rate, she's full of questions and, most important, all ears.

Screen Gems

Take a few cues from the beautylicious bad girls of the silver screen. Carmen Jones smoldered. She scorched Joe (the very fine Harry Belafonte) so badly, Papa went mental wondering what else he could do to please her. A word of caution, because we did see the end of the movie: Although you want to drive Brother a touch crazy (in the figurative sense, of course) you don't want to drive him to a crime of passion. Intensity, passion, fun, and great sex are the goals here. Permanent chill at Forest Lawn is not. With that said, let's take a few notes from Miss Carmen and a few other beautylicious bad girls (BBGs). Learn sexy tactics that are so hot they'll have to call the fire department on you. Make him feel the burn.

> *BBG:* Carmen Jones (Dorothy Dandridge) from *Carmen Jones*
> *BBG move:* Hiding out in a shabby Chicago hotel room, Carmen had just given herself a pedicure, while Joe was droning on about life on the run. She languidly raised her leg in Joe's direction and drawled, "Blow on 'em, Sugar. Makes 'em dry faster."
> *Lesson for you:* Take a mundane grooming act and make it so intimate it's criminal.

> *BBG:* Sparkle's older, beautiful sister, Sister (Lonette McKee) from *Sparkle*
> *BBG move:* Sister always stole the show by breaking away from the group to wiggle and preen. The crowd, especially the men, would eat it up.
> *Lesson for you:* Strut your stuff with confidence.

BBG: Nola Darling (Tracy Camilla Johns) from *She's Gotta Have It*

BBG move: Nola was unashamedly dating three radically different guys who obviously appealed to different aspects of her personality. She was so cocksure of herself that she invited them all to dinner.

Lesson for you: You're free and single. Hang out with a variety of guys. Tell the brothers up front and let the world know there is no shame in your game!

BBG: Shug (Margaret Avery) from *The Color Purple*

BBG move: Shug showered everyone from Mister to Celie with attention and made them feel special.

Lesson for you: Flirt with everybody—man, woman, beast, vegetable, or mineral.

BBG: Tracy Chambers (Diana Ross) from *Mahogany*

BBG move: While in the unemployment office, Tracy created a scene about trying to get her old man back, which helped Brian (Billy Dee Williams) grab the attention of potential voters in his run for alderman and in the process cemented his interest in and ardor for her.

Lesson for you: Support the Brother. You've been checking him out and you have some idea of what's important to him. Share his interests with humor and creativity. Simply seize the moment and improvise.

Meet Market

There are men all over the place and there are probably more than a couple for you. Don't miss out on someone fabulous because you're wedded to a certain type. Sure, we all deserve a dreamboat with Denzel Washington's charm and charisma, Miles Davis's sartorial sense, Sam Jackson's cool, and Boris Kodjoe's chiseled good looks coupled with a Harvard MBA and JD, but what are the odds of that happening? And guess what, the odds are even lower when all you do is go from home to work and work to home. Get out, explore, and enjoy yourself in the process. Leave no stone unturned in the pursuit of men.

MACK ATTACK

You're meandering down aisle five at the supermarket when you see a vision of utter fineness squeezing the Charmin. Or while riding the subway to work you look over the lifestyle section of *USA Today* and gaze into a pair of the most beautiful and kindest brown eyes you've ever seen. What to do? Should you depend on him to make the first move? Baby, reverse the tables and throw him a line, but not just any smarmy line. Reach for something clever yet simple. So simple, in fact, that it is greatly underused. The pickup line that works every time: *Hi!*

FEAR FACTOR

Shake things up. Get out of your comfort zone and take a walk on the wild side. Pry yourself away from the frat house and go to a dance given by the Loyal Order of the Moose and Elks. Shy? Push yourself to make eye contact and speak to the first guy who catches your eye on your way to the store. Swearing blindly that you only date guys your age? Well it's time to swing a young buck or an old school baller for fun and variety. So what if you have your Ph.D., play like Claudine and wink at the sanitation man. The idea is to do whatever scares you the most about dating; con-

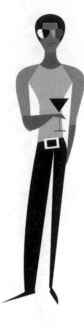

front it head-on. Whenever you hear yourself saying, "I would never . . ." well, that's the very thing you need to do. Within limits of course. You won't get my blessing to walk toward Mr. "I just got out of lockdown" under the guise of having a new experience. Already worried that the men you turn up won't be right? Pshaw! Remember this: There are no guarantees in love and that is the guarantee. So get out there and be bold, beautiful, and brave.

TURN ON YOUR GAYDAR

A few scary facts: A recently released report from the Centers for Disease Control revealed that 63 percent of all women with HIV/AIDS were black. And of the 63 percent, 38 percent contracted HIV/AIDS from sexual contact. Ahem, no one can afford to keep her head in the sand about a bisexual, "Down Low" (DL), or homosexual (or drug-abusing) boyfriend. Don't always go by looks. Mr. Thug lovin' can be just as much of a problem as the "particular" doctor. Of course, there are no sure-fire ways of telling if your man's a switch-hitter if you don't catch him on the downstroke, but there are a few signs floating around that should make you say hmm. . . .

1. Can identify last season's Versace shoes and duds for women and scornfully mentions them.
2. Loves the following divas: Diana, Patti, Judy, and Barbra and divas in training like Lil' Kim and Destiny's Child. Note there is a difference between appreciation (knowing and liking a few songs) and love (knowing the song, its history, and why, when, and where the diva first sang it. Also can imitate the diva's mannerisms). The dead

giveaway: The Brother who puts his world on hold when said diva is in town and buys tickets to each performance. He's been doing that since age sixteen.

3. Hates gays and has a penchant for name-calling. Methinks he doth protest too much.

4. Has an overprotective best friend or frat brother. You know, the one who always tells you he knows Lamar better than you do.

5. Is secretive about parts of his life.

6. Is a barrel of laughs at the museum but mysteriously clams up when you two are within twenty feet of the bedroom.

All jokes aside, in matters of the heart and health you must follow your gut and step off, or at the very least use a condom. Don't be ashamed to employ Mom's old maxim: If it walks like a duck, quacks like a duck, and looks like a duck, it's a duck. Act accordingly.

COFFEE, TEA, OR LEAVE

You're lying next to a 220-pound hunk. Last night he was a hunk in the best definition of the term; now, at 2 A.M., he's been demoted to hunk of junk. After you've been staring at the ceiling for what seems like forever, your little mind is fast at work on trying to exit stage left. Not to worry, sit bolt upright and declare, "Omigosh, I've got to get the house ready for Aunt Clara!" Call a car service, gather up your things, and run. However, if the hunk turns out to be a hunk of burning love and you want to hang on and out, don't go needy with a wheedling, "Whatcha doing? I would love for you to spend the rest of the day with me!" Go the cool, calm, and collected route and tell him what's on your agenda. Dreamily say, "I am going to check out the best of the 'Black Exploitation' movies at the Film Forum." If he is game, tell him a world of gators, girls, and fly brims awaits him. If he gives you the shaft, don't take offense but take the hint and your clothes and go!

THE MOANING AFTER

If Saturday you two were kicking it and Sunday you feel kicked to the curb, don't cry, don't pout or go ballistic. Just answer the following questions honestly. Did Lover sign any contract saying he owed you a call within twenty-four hours? Would the case fly with Judge Mablean? No! All right, for the love of Prada, please avoid the "For Colored Girls" overwrought soliloquy route. If you can handle a phone call without attitude and drama, why not place the "thanks, I had fun" call. The bottom line: Whatever Bro's intentions or feelings, they aren't likely to change, so why drain your energy or waste perfectly good talent?

HOW TO HANDLE A BREAKUP

Homie has given you your walking papers, and boy does it hurt. The only thing keeping you from committing a major

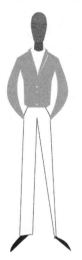

felony is the fact that the orange jumpsuit is really so unbecoming . . . Well, what's a girl to do when she's forced to go solo? Have a celebration, damn it! Pick a day and call it "A little sad but still fab" day. And on that glorious day, throw yourself a major pity party. Stay in the bed with a pint of Häagen-Dazs Dulce de Leche at your side. Pop your favorite tearjerker into the VCR; it's a good time for *Imitation of Life* or *Brian's Song.* Lie in bed and just cry . . . about Brian, Pecola, and yourself. Once you finish crying, take a nap. Get on the bat phone to your friends and wail, "Why?" fifty million times. It's your day, so your friends will listen and coo sympathetically and give good advice without telling you they're sick to death of this story. After another outburst of tears it should be dinnertime. Make it champagne and Popeye's spicy chicken. While chowing down—I promise—you'll miraculously start to see that ole Loverboy was a jerk or he really wasn't for you. Go with that feeling for a minute. Savor it. Write down his pros and cons if you wish. Don't call him for his version. Go from the list of his pros and cons to making your own. Go over what you have to live for and what therefore makes you so beautylicious. What do you know—it's bedtime and tomorrow should be easier to face.

SONGS IN THE KEY OF B FLAT

A breakup hurts like hell. Whatever stage of the breakup you're in, there are a few tunes to wail to.

Pining for the Loss of Love

It's clear the relationship is on the limp-along plan, but Mr. Lover Lover does have a few redeeming qualities (honestly?!) and you're trying to hang on.

"Foolish," Ashanti
"If Only for One Night," Brenda Russell (she's got the
    plaintive, one-more-for-the-road sound)
"The Long and Winding Road," George Benson
"Just to Keep You Satisfied," Marvin Gaye
"I'm Catching Hell," Natalie Cole
"Fallin'," Alicia Keys

Dropped and Hurtin'

Scoundrel. Cad. Bounder. Used to be my man. Yep, you're certifiably bitter and blue.

"Not Going to Cry," Mary J. Blige
"I Can't Make You Love Me," Bonnie Raitt
"Ain't No Way," Aretha Franklin
"Unbreak My Heart," Toni Braxton
"Thin Line Between Love and Hate," The Persuaders
"My Mistake," Diana Ross and Marvin Gaye
"Good Morning Heartache," Billie Holiday
"What's Love Got to Do with It," Tina Turner
"Love Don't Live Here Anymore," Rose Royce

The Dawn of Optimism

One morning you poke your head out from under the covers and in the blinding sunlight you feel like it's all going to be just fine. Your ideal Brotherman's out there and you're ready to resume your search for him. Begin humming "The Man I Love."

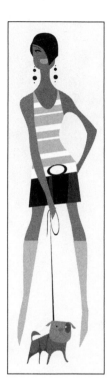

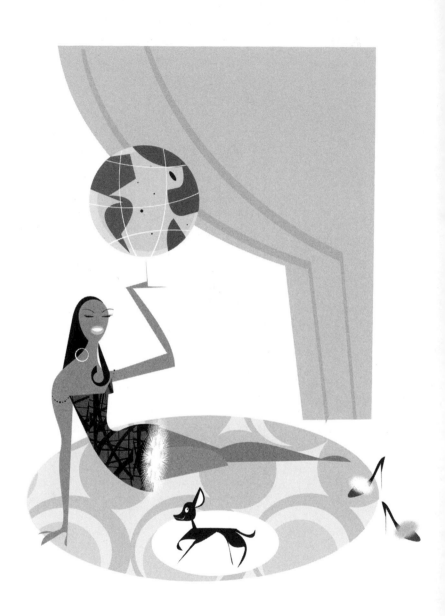

Chapter Ten

Luxe Life

*Take care of the luxuries and the
necessities will take care of themselves.*
—DOROTHY PARKER

Splurge, Baby, Splurge!

What's the use of taking up space on this great earth if you don't partake of all of the beauty, riches, and fun life has to offer? Cultivate your voluptuary interests. Indulge! Quit boring your dates by ordering rabbit food; have a juicy piece of filet mignon and don't apologize to him or yourself about it. Gather posies for your office or call FTD and have them deliver roses to you on the job. Bottom line, find out what makes the ordinary extraordinary for you. Consider the venerable designer Coco Chanel's maxim: "Luxury must be comfortable, otherwise it is not luxury." What makes you feel good?

Take a page from Miles Davis, who lived a luxurious life. The singular trumpeter defined luxury as whatever appealed to his finely tuned sense of aesthetics. It could be anything from the sleek lines of his Ferrari, butter-soft Italian leather furniture, the sharp crease in his tailor-made nun cloth trousers, or the joys of putting together a gourmet meal. For Miles it was a real appreciation of the product. The precise workmanship, the finely spun silk, now, that was the real turn-on.

Think of the innovative trumpet player and learn about what you like and define why it's fabulous for you. That's not Puffy's job. If you enjoy the experience of drinking tea, the luxury may be in having a nice steaming pot of Darjeeling as opposed to your usual Tetley fix. Besides, the beautylicious babe knows that a designer name doesn't necessarily mean luxury. Sometimes it just means overpriced. Of course, in some instances, most notably diamonds and fur, there are political and moral issues to consider. Ms. Beautylicious isn't one to profit off pain, or remain willfully ignorant of the various issues. She does, however, remain open-minded.

Luxe for Less

Some wise soul, probably Mom, once said, "You should fill your life with little luxuries." I always thought she made that up so that I could get over the fact that I wasn't getting a pony (a real luxury, uhm, okay, a stupid expenditure for a family in the city), but the dear girl has a point. Here is a list of little luxuries that will make you feel as rich as Oprah:

1. *Invest in elegant stationery.* You should have classic note cards made of good stock at your disposal. Visit Cartier, Tiffany, Smythson of Bond Street, or Dempsey & Carroll for chic correspondence.
2. *Get a massage.* You can go to a swank spa or to the Y for a masseuse.
3. *Take a cooking course.* Look to a culinary institute in your area.
4. *Learn a new language. Parlez-vouz français* at the local community college or by using some Berlitz tapes and teaching yourself.
5. *Replace your wire hangers* with wooded and feminine padded hangers.
6. *Stock up on lovely linen and cotton napkins.* Use them when you eat instead of paper towels. Troll

vintage stores and flea markets for beautiful
and inexpensive finds.

7. *Buy a piece of art.* It doesn't matter if it's a
poster, a painting from the dude down the
block, or an original Bearden; just buy
something that makes your heart soar
when you look at it.

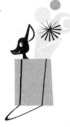

8. *Find a sumptuous meal in a cookbook and create it for
yourself.* Step out of your comfort zone of chicken and
greens and learn to make something different, like a
foreign dish or an entree that has always made your
mouth water, like shepherd's pie. Look to a cookbook like
Nigella Bites by Nigella Lawson (Hyperion) for great
recipes.

9. *Jazz up a mundane food item.* Hit the specialty grocery for
tasty items like honey infused with ginger or a dazzling
array of teas.

10. *Treat your friends and family.* Splurge on a manicure for
Ma, Sis, and your best friend.

Diamonds

The little rock may say *forever,* in terms of love, prestige, and
value, but, Dollface, how well do you really know your diamonds? Let's face it, we all know about the same three things: it
needs to come out of a blue box when we get engaged, you
shouldn't need a microscope to see it, and there is such a thing
as too much—as seen on most rappers. Well, that ain't gonna cut
it. (And by the way, the only thing that cuts a diamond is another diamond.) Let's get down to basics: The diamond is made
of pure or nearly pure carbon. It possesses three spectacular
qualities, the first being the power of light reflection. The cut

diamond gathers light within itself and sends back a blinding brilliance. Second, it is the purest gemstone in that it is composed of one element. (Are you starting to get why you should have stayed awake for chemistry and earth science?) And third, it is the hardest substance known to man.

You can also learn from your jeweler. If you're a big jewelry fan, your jeweler needs to be picked with the same utmost care that you used to select a hairdresser. In other words, the ice man needs to be trustworthy and blessed with a sharp and discerning eye. Ask around for recommendations or take a minute and audition a few until you find one with whom you're comfortable. Now, the ice man should cometh with a few simple truths, the first being that bigger isn't always better. Yep, diamonds are sold by weight and measured in carats and expressed in decimals. To make it real for you: Five carats equals a gram—big even for Liz Taylor and P. Diddy, while your baby niece's diamond studs (unless she's the offspring of a baller) are probably a point or one-one-hundredth of a carat. Size alone means nothing if the stone lacks brilliance, purity, and high-grade color. Simply put, it's wise to consider the four Cs before you try to bring the bling:

Cut: Determines the brilliance of a diamond. To get serious bling-bling, the diamond cutter places each of the stone's facets, which act as light-dispensing mirrors, in exact geometric relation to one another. Of course, this is the goal that top jewelers "reach for." Many lesser jewelers will cut the stone to maximize size.

Clarity: The fewer the flaws, the clearer and more brilliant the ice. The clarity grades range from *Fl* for flawless to *I* for imperfect.

Color: The more colorless the diamond, the greater its rarity and value. Diamonds are color-graded ranging from *D*, colorless, to *Z*, light yellow. A little color isn't a deal breaker, but a rock that's as foggy as London town is a no-go.

Carat weight is simply the gemologist's measure of a diamond's size.

DICEY ICE

Diamonds may be a girl's best friend, but not if they have blood on them. Our sisters and brothers are being mutilated and in some instances killed because of the rebel guerrilla groups that control the African diamond mines of Sierra Leone, Tanzania, and Angola. The diamonds from these regions are referred to as conflict diamonds. While conflict diamonds are anywhere from 5 to 15 percent of the international diamond trade, they are in circulation all over the world.

How do you guard against buying a conflict diamond and unwittingly supporting murderous regimes in the motherland? You really can't. There is no way you can purchase a diamond with 100 percent assurance that it is not a conflict diamond. You can, however, make a lot of noise and let the jeweler know you're concerned about the situation in Africa. Ask for diamonds from Botswana, Namibia, South Africa, or Canada. The trade association of jewelers, Jewelers of America, and the World Diamond Council are currently working closely with Congress on a proposed bill, the Clean Diamond Act, which has passed in the House but not in the Senate, to put controls into place, and on a global bill, the Kimberley Process, which will curtail and control the world market. Educate yourself on the topic and locate clean diamond dealers by reading the Amnesty International site (www.amnestyusa.org/diamonds). Look for synthetic diamonds. Not your mama's cubic zirconias, the newest synthetic diamond is virtually indistinguishable from the real thing. Gemesis and Apollo Diamonds are the two companies leading the way, creating ice that costs 10 to 50 percent less than the naturals. How good are the dubious diamonds? Let's just say, De Beers is disgusted. The stones made the Gemesis way can only be detected with very expensive machines (the kind used in international gem labs) and the Apollo diamond can't be detected at all. Or you can take a stand like India. Arie and Alicia Keys and just say no dice to ice. Rediscover the beauty of your birth-month gem, along with spectacular sparklers like the sapphire, ruby, or emerald.

Champagne: The Elixir of the Fabulous

Nothing says *swell elegance* like champagne. It's effervescent and brings out a certain joie de vivre, hmm, sort of like you! The bubbles, the sweetly giddy feeling (the carbon and oxygen released through the bubbles allow the alcohol to be quickly absorbed by the bloodstream), and the fact that champagne goes with almost any food make it downright sexy. The grandest of libations, champagne should not be relegated to celebrations. The cork should be popped *just because*.

Back in the day, the bubbly of choice for Eartha, Diahann, Josephine P., and the smart set was Dom Perignon. Today, Puffy almost single-handedly has made Cristal the drink of a new generation. Here are the frothy facts on the world's most festive drink. Champagne is technically a wine that hails from the Champagne region of France, which is ninety miles northeast of Paris. Got it? If the fizzy juice comes from California, Spain, Italy, etc., it's referred to as sparkling wine.

What exactly should you look for in your champagne? The same qualities that your man and friends should have: character, flavor, balance, and harmony. It should not be acidic (champagne hasn't aged) or rough. The bubbles, however, should be small and plentiful and the taste should be smooth with a biscuity, nutty, or slightly fruity taste.

While His Diddyness continues to make what amounts to unpaid advertising of Cristal, have you ever wondered what makes Cristal better than, let's say, André, aside from the price tag? What you need to know is that Dom P and Cristal are considered prestige cuvées in that they epitomize the best of a particular champagne house (which makes and sells the bubbly using its own vineyard). The cuvées are produced in small quantities, and it is their rarity that determines the high price. There are two hundred fifty houses, but the four most popular houses in the States are Moët & Chandon, which is the biggest and the home of Dom P; Louis Roederer, the most exclusive and the home of Cristal; Perrier-Jouët, home of Belle Époque (the pretty floral bottle); and Veuve Clicquot Ponsardin, home of La Grande Dame Brut. And, while Sean John claims that Cristal doesn't cause hangovers, the truth is that no champagne will cause a hangover if you drink responsibly (i.e., don't guzzle down every bottle in sight) and if you drink only champagne and don't mix it with other common spirits.

CARE AND SERVING OF THE BUBBLY

+ Champagne, more than other wines, is sensitive to light and temperature, so keep it stored in a cool place (like your cabinet, if you don't have a wine cellar) in its box.
+ The preferred (and also the quickest) way to chill champagne is by letting it sit in a bucket of ice and water, but you can chill it in the fridge for up to two hours. No long stints in the fridge, as that will suppress the bouquet and the cork might stick.
+ When opening the bottle, remember that the cork can eas-

ily turn into a deadly weapon if the bottle isn't opened properly. Take care to remove the foil, the wire cage, and the metal cap at the top of the cork. With the bottle on a stable surface like a table or countertop, gently turn and rock the cork while covering it with your hand. When you feel the cork trying to push out, hold it back a bit to allow the gas to escape slowly.

✦ Think of pouring the champagne as a sensual delight. First pour a little into your glass, and watch and listen as the bubbles dance. On the second pouring, fill the glass until it is three-quarters full and enjoy the color and the way the bubbles tickle your nose. Now bring the glass to your lips and sip.

✦ The appropriate glass for champagne is a straight-sided flute or a tulip glass.

✦ If you have leftover champagne, drink it! Of course, if the bottle is more than half full and you've passed your drinking limits, simply recork the bottle or invest in a champagne stopper, so that you can save the bubbles.

FIZZY LINGO

Cuvée: The best juice from the best grape.

Brut: The classic style of bubbly; dry (anywhere from zero to fifteen grams of sugar).

Demi-Sec: A semisweet champagne that goes wonderfully with desserts and spicy food.

Rosé: Grapes are blended with a darker grape like the pinot noir for a slightly pinkish blush.

Jeroboam: A large bottle equivalent to four bottles of champagne. But by no means the econo size or price!

Magnum: A large bottle equivalent to two bottles of champagne, best for six or more people.

Split: A small bottle equivalent to two small glasses of

champagne. Sip it with a straw for
fun!

Vintage: The grapes used in a particular
year are of excellent quality.

Nonvintage: Designates champagne that
is a blend of wines from different
years, thus it is less expensive.
Nonvintage is 90 percent of the
champagne that's sipped.

Fur

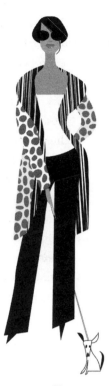

Undeniably glamorous, fur has always been
an entrance maker. And boy oh boy, can a
diva work it. Think of Bessie Smith drag-
ging a full-length mink behind her as she
sings the blues; Josephine Baker shimmying
the night away in a silver fox with nothing
on underneath it, mesmerizing Ernest Hemingway; or Cleopatra
Jones kicking butt in a sassy rabbit chubby jacket. You see, Ma
was right about the fur being for special occasions; it works with
whatever you deem special. Fur is the ultimate glamour accou-
trement and an expensive one, so consider the following before
you succumb to the first pretty fur you see:

+ Look at your lifestyle and what you want to use the fur for.
+ Figure out your budget. The cost includes more than the
  actual purchase of the coat. Remember, it has to be stored
  and cleaned.
+ Find a reputable furrier. Like your jeweler, your furrier is
  now an auxiliary member of Team Me.
+ Think about your figure, but keep an open mind. While

there are no real rules about what fur is best with what figure type, know that long-haired furs like fox or coyote will
add a bit of heft, and that floor-length, long-haired furs
will envelop a short or small frame.

✦ Try on everything that you like regardless of price. You'll
be surprised at what looks good.

✦ Be prepared to drop lots of cash on chinchilla and sable skin,
for they are considered the Rolls-Royce of furs. Chinchilla is
extremely fragile; it will tear if left hanging on a hanger.
And, most important, it takes many of the little fellows to
make a coat. Sable and chinchilla are best used as trim.

✦ Think mink. Mink offers the first-time fur buyer versatility
as an everyday coat and a dress coat, and it doesn't shed.
Plus, the short-haired fur makes it flattering to a variety of
figures. Don't overlook sheared beaver as a trendsetting alternative to mink.

LEGENDARY FUR WEARERS

Back in the day, Blackglama mink ran a hugely popular and
iconic ad campaign that featured some of the most glamorous
women in the world swathed in their opulent furs. Six Dolls
added a little soul and sass to the pelts. "Who becomes a legend
most?" Lena Horne, Diana Ross, Leontyne Price, DeeDee
Bridgewater, Eartha Kitt, and Diahann Carroll, of course.

CONSIDER THE MINK'S CIVIL RIGHTS

Fur sports an NPC (not politically correct) rating in certain
quarters. PETA (People for the Ethical Treatment of Animals),
which counts actress Traci Bingham as a supporter, believes essentially that animals have rights and they are not ours to use
for food, clothing, entertainment, or experimentation. Be clear:
In PETA's world vision, one doesn't wear leather, eat burgers,
spritz crawly things with bug spray, or go big-game hunting.

The tactics PETA has used to make its point have included everything from terrorizing fur wearers by taunting them in public to throwing paint on fur coats. Often the PETA folks cede their moral ground by violating someone else's civil rights in favor of the dearly departed mink, fox, or rabbit's rights. While their tactics and thought process can be downright fascist, most animal lovers and lovers of life can understand their point. Can't we all just get along in God's country? Well, we can all try. If you're still chowing down on steaks and pining for Manolo's alligator pumps, you may need to consider more of an animal welfare approach to fur, which means it's okay as long as humane guidelines are followed.

It's your call. And, of course, if all else fails there's nothing like a fabulous faux fur or a billowy down coat (not as chic) to keep you warm.

Room Service

Splurge and turn your home into a pleasure palace. It's easy and it's expensive, but you're worth it!

Flowers

Ahh ... little Lotus Blossom, get rid of the notion that flowers are only for Valentine's Day, Easter, and home-going services. Flowers are living art. They add color, beauty, and a touch of fragrance to your abode. Stop and really smell the roses. Cultivate a few floral fantasies and fulfill them. Think of yourself as a Cotton Club showgirl with a dressing room full of flowers from various stage-door johnnies and fill your bedroom with white roses. (Note: This one can be used as an intimidation tactic on Boyfriend!) Re-create a Caribbean island with an explosion of vibrant blossoms. Whatever gets you going to the florist or the garden. Consider these tips on when to choose flowers, how to arrange them, and how to care for them.

The beautylicious babe is always captivated by what are called "mass flowers." They are generally round and full-faced with one flower per stem. The perennial favorites are:

> *Roses:* Look for buds open or flowers tight-centered with some leaves on stem. *Special treat:* Immerse them in a small amount of boiling water (no more than one-quarter of a cup), which preserves the blooms and opens the buds. Follow with lukewarm water up to the first leaves or stems and add two tablespoons of salt.
>
> *Tulips:* Look for buds showing color. *Special treat:* Place them in a small amount of warm water with a half-teaspoon of sugar, to keep them perky longer.
>
> *Irises, daisies, carnations, gerbera daisies, and sunflowers:* Look for flowers open and stems firm. *Special treat:* Keep 'em, ahem, daisy fresh with three drops of peppermint oil in a quart of water.

In choosing a vase, be inventive. Anything goes, as long as it doesn't upstage the blooms. A few stylish choices include:

- ✦ Crystal
- ✦ Enamel household pitchers
- ✦ Galvanized steel buckets
- ✦ Colored glass bottles
- ✦ Mismatched glass jars

Don't let the vase engulf the flowers. The tallest flower should be two and a half times the height of an upright vase.

For a modern and sophisticated look, cut the stems of roses or other heavy-bloomed flowers like peonies and camellias two inches below the head. Put them together in a silver-plated mint julep cup or a small glass vase.

Arranging Grace

After you've chosen about twenty-one stems (always an odd number for optimum balance, and a mixture of bloom and filler flowers—you know, the leafy ferns and baby's breath) in some stunning color combination, choose a medium-height vase. Half-fill the vase with water. Crisscross the stems of the filler flowers as you put them in the vase. This creates a grid to hold the other flowers in place. Start at the outside rim with the shortest and smallest flowers and work toward the center, adding flowers in ascending height to create a very loose triangle. Stand back and look at the arrangement as you go along.

Baby Your Buds

Keep flowers well fed and relatively wilt-proof by removing leaves that go in the water, so that the flowers can drink up and the water doesn't look like a cesspool. Cut flower stems diagonally at the base, except tulips, which are cut straight. Display your flowers in a cool, draft-free place. Add water daily, and change the water after several days.

Candles in the Lair

Candles create a mood and are also very soothing. They can light up any room and they come in a myriad of shapes, colors, and scents. Choose according to your mood. The *votive* (looks bite-size) when placed in a candle holder creates a warm glow. *Pillars* (large blocks of wax in oval or rectangular shapes) are great for long-lasting burn and scents. If you're going for a candlelight dinner, opt for *tapers*, which are unscented, so as not to conflict with the delicious smell of your cooking. Nothing is more delightful than a few decorative fragrant candles to lightly scent your living space. Now, not every scented candle actually provides an appreciable scent once it's lit. Whether the scent will waft throughout the room depends greatly on the amount of essential oils and fragrance that are imbued in the candle. Six candle brands (in a range of prices averaging fifteen to sixty dollars) that pass the sniff test: Archipelago, L'Occitane, Ergo, Votivo, Diptyque, and Rigaud. On the move? Bring a piece of home with you in a small votive candle in your favorite scent.

Be responsible about burning candles so that you don't set your pad on fire. A few tips:

- ✦ Keep lit candles away from flammable materials and accessories like curtains, bedding, shower curtains, and so forth.
- ✦ Always extinguish candles before going to bed.
- ✦ Never burn candles without candleholders.
- ✦ Keep candles at least one inch away from each other so shorter candles will not melt into the sides of taller candles.
- ✦ Always clean wax residue from candleholders.
- ✦ Never leave candles unattended or where children or pets could be injured.

Dream Sheets

It is estimated that you spend a third of your life in bed. Why not spend at least a third of the third swathed in sinfully soft sheets? Bed down in cotton sheets with a high thread count. The thread count simply refers to how many threads per inch are used to weave a sheet. Most of us spend our time tossing and turning on 180-thread-count sheets, a cotton or cotton/polyester blend called percale, which is a standard weave. But as the thread count gets higher—think 250 and above—the sheets become softer and last longer.

Cotton is king because it is cooler to sleep on, keeps the clammy feeling down since the fiber directs moisture away from your skin, and is less likely to stain because it releases dirt easily when wet. The sheets that dreams are made of usually come from France, think Porthault and Frette, and Italy, the home of Pratesi. These lines are coveted because they use Egyptian cotton (the longest cotton fibers make for stronger, more sumptuous linen), for the high thread count, usually 300 and up, and for the exquisite craftsmanship—hand-embroidered edges or touches of lace. Yes, you can blow as much *dinero* on the sheets as you would on your rent, but the good news is that you can expect the European sheets to last you at least ten to twenty years. On the other hand, you can still enjoy a divine sleeping experience and have enough money to pay the phone bill. Snuggle up to pima cotton, which also has long fibers and is grown in the United States, Peru, and Australia. When you see the term *supima*, know that we're now talking about superior pima, the best cotton the United States has to offer. While you're saving up for Pratesi, don't overlook brands like Martha Stewart, Wamsutta, Ralph Lauren, or those of your favorite department store for cozy sheets. Or order sheets online at www.domesticbin.com or www.bluefly.com for great savings.

Chocolate Goodies

The sweetest extravagance in candy land, chocolate is one of the simplest delights in the world and one of the sexiest.

Beautylicious moment: Pallie Marcita and I were prowling through Neiman Marcus when we happened upon the chocolate. Of course, we had to buy some truffles. As we were strolling down Rodeo Drive we both bit into one. What happened next is a testament to the power of chocolate. We were actually moaning and sighing in ecstasy after each bite—loudly. Ridiculous! Years later, we still reminisce about the absolute best truffle. Who would think a piece of chocolate could move you to great heights? Er, scientists, that's who. It seems that chocolate contains phenylethylamine (PEA), a chemical your brain secretes when you are in love, hence its reputation as an aphrodisiac. And guess what, chocolate is also good for you because it acts as an antioxidant. Dark chocolate seems to lower the risk of heart disease, lung cancer, and asthma.

Great! The medical community is cool with cocoa. Now you must figure out why you should spend more than seventy-five cents on candy. Chocolate, like shoes, is all about *your* taste. No one can tell you what you should like, but there are some general criteria to consider in order to determine whether a chocolate is fine enough for you. First, look at the pieces to make sure that they are a consistent color with a satin sheen and that they are free of air bubbles and blemishes. A dull shade generally says that the chocolate hasn't been stored or handled properly. Sniff your candy. Fine chocolates are made of the highest-quality cocoa beans and a high percentage of cocoa butter; thus they should have a fresh deep aroma and not the sugary scent that is often associated with preservatives and, *quelle horreur,* artificial flavoring. Naturally, you must taste the chocolate to determine both the flavor and the texture. Freshly made bonbons have a very intense but refined flavor. The candy should "snap" when you bite into it. When tasting a piece of chocolate, let it melt against the roof of your mouth to feel the texture. It should feel velvety smooth. The master chocolatiers insist that fine chocolate will satisfy your craving with just one or two pieces because of the intensity of the aroma, texture, and flavor. We all know that the beautylicious babe is just getting started, so indulge and enjoy. But remember, if you can't eat your chocolate within a week or two, you can refrigerate or freeze it. Simply roll the pieces in several layers of plastic wrap and place them in an airtight container to prevent wetness. Defrost at room temperature without unwrapping.

Three haute chocolates you must try or make somebody buy: La Maison du Chocolat (www.lamaisonduchocolat.com), Teuscher (www.teuscherchocolate.com), and Richart (www. richart-chocolates.com). Or look to your local chocolatier.

SOME LUXURIOUS WAYS TO ENJOY YOUR CHOCOLATE

C'mon, why limit yourself to Hershey bars and Nesquik? Discover the delicious lure of cocoa by changing your setting, your mind-set, and the chocolate!

+ Make chocolate-covered strawberries and enjoy a dessert *à deux* or alone with a glass of champagne.
+ Pretend your apartment or his is in the Plaza Hotel, turn back the bed sheets, and put a coin-size piece of the best chocolate on the pillow. Place the rest of the chocolate in a small beautiful bowl or a kitschy dish next to the bed.
+ Drizzle a bit of chocolate liqueur on your ice cream, cake, brownie, or beau and eat up. Or pour two shot glasses' worth into your nightly coffee for a warm and incredibly yummy drink.
+ Whip up the most sinful version of hot chocolate known to mankind:

Sinful Hot Chocolate

2½ CUPS WHOLE MILK

¼ CUP BOILING WATER

¼ CUP GRANULATED SUGAR

2 OUNCES DARK BITTERSWEET CHOCOLATE (TRY LINDT),
    FINELY SLICED WITH A BREAD KNIFE

¼ CUP COCOA POWDER (TRY GODIVA)

WHIPPED CREAM

In a two-quart saucepan, combine the milk, water, and sugar and bring to a boil over medium heat. Add the chopped chocolate and cocoa, bring to a boil again, then reduce heat while whisking until chocolate and cocoa are dissolved and the mixture has thickened. Reduce the heat to low. Add a heaping dollop of whipped cream to each serving and enjoy!

Makes four 6-ounce cups of hot chocolate

The Biggest Luxury of All . . . Okay, Kitten, pop quiz: What is the biggest luxury of all? Hit the back of the class if you think it is the Hope Diamond, a Franck Muller watch, a Bentley, Rolls-Royce or whatever the latest plaything of the rich and famous is. The beautylicious babe instinctively knows that the most luxurious thing in the world doesn't have a price tag—because peace of mind is priceless.

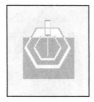

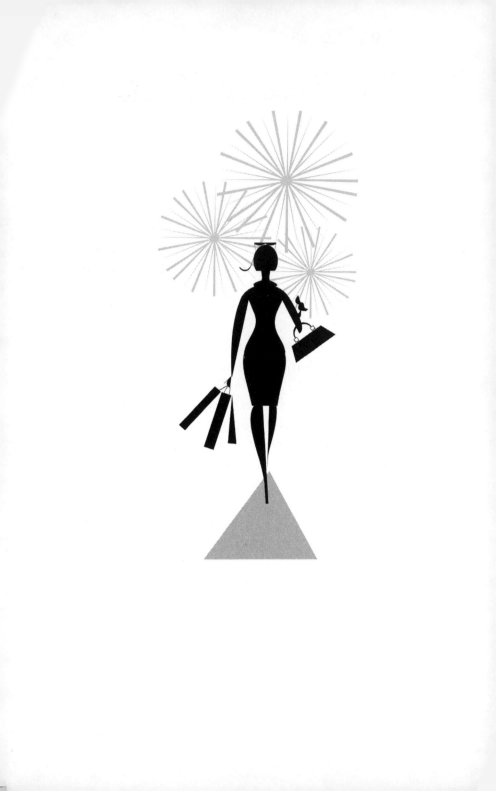

The Fabulous Finale

Well, Cupcake, our romp replete with boys, bubbles, baubles, and Blahniks has come to an end. Ohh, no, maybe a new beginning. So let's raise our champagne glass (you do have a bit left, right?) and say "Cheers" to the moment. Because in this moment the beautylicious babe (that's you, Toots) knows that she can do or be what she wants. And that, my dears, is the raison d'être of this little tome. So let's stand tall in our Manolos or Marabou Slippers and recite the Beautylicious Oath. (Sort of like a recap, but treat it like an affirmation!!)

I, [your name], am a beautylicious babe. I know the world is mine for the taking. Thanks to God, I possess many gifts, including my unique beauty, sensual body, and fierce intellect. I am committed to the love and betterment of me—through learning, exercise, and taking risks. I walk a path of love and grace, which precludes me from being rude, ill-tempered, or obnoxious. I am kind and loving to people, animals, and the surrounding world. I follow my heart, be it in romance or the prospect of a new career. I am not afraid to fall 'cause I know I will get back up. I deserve whatever I want out of life and I thank God for the moxie to go after it. I know I rule! Toodles!

About the Author

Jenyne Raines is the former associate beauty editor at *Essence* and has more than ten years' experience in writing about black beauty and style. Her articles have appeared in *InStyle, Vibe, Heart & Soul, Mode, Girl,* and *Weight Watchers.* Raines has also contributed to three books: *SoulStyle: Black Women Defining Fashion, Tenderheaded: A Comb-bending Collection of Hair Stories,* and *Essence Total Makeover.* She has consulted for leading beauty companies, including Revlon, Clairol, Black Opal, and PhytoSpecific.